How to Prevent And Reverse Heart Diseases

And even Avoid Bye Pass

© 2013 by **Prem Chhatwani**

Income Disclaimer

This document contains business strategies, marketing methods and other business advice that, regardless of my own results and experience, may not produce the same results (or any results) for you. I make absolutely no guarantee, expressed or implied, that by following the advice below you will make any money or improve current profits, as there are several factors and variables that come into play regarding any given business.

Primarily, results will depend on the nature of the product or business model, the conditions of the marketplace, the experience of the individual, and situations and elements that are beyond your control.

As with any business endeavor, you assume all risk related to investment and money based on your own discretion and at your own potential expense.

Liability Disclaimer

By reading this document, you assume all risks associated with using the advice given below, with a full understanding that you, solely, are responsible for anything that may occur as a result of putting this information into action in any way, and regardless of your interpretation of the advice.

You further agree that our company cannot be held responsible in any way for the success or failure of your business as a result of the information presented below. It is your responsibility to conduct your own due diligence regarding the safe and successful operation of your business if you intend to apply any of our information in any way to your business operations.

Terms of Use

You are given a non-transferable, "personal use" license to this product. You cannot distribute it or share it with other individuals.

Also, there are no resale rights or private label rights granted when purchasing this document. In other words, it's for your own personal use only.

Table of Contents

The pathway of blood flow through the heart

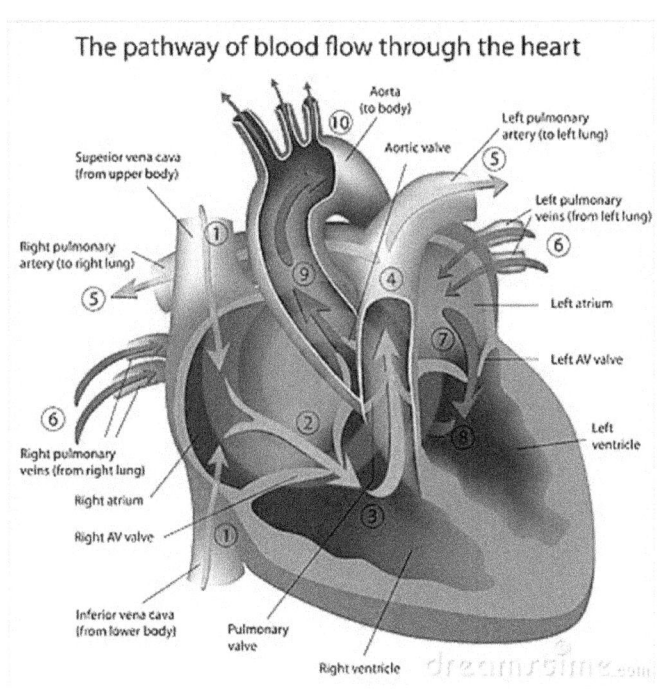

My Personal Journey

Over the years I had lot of interest in Alternate Therapies, including Homoeopathic medicines, Herbal and Ayurvedic treatments for various diseases.

At age 28 I got hit by Asthma. My Dad had Asthma for years and I had witnessed his sufferings. So I kind of inherited the disease but at a later age than as a child.

My Mom had heart problems but she actually died of Cancer in her late fifties.

With family history like that, I did not know what to expect in my older years. At age of around 50, with slightly high Cholesterol (230-240) and still using inhalers like Albuterol Sulfate and Cortisone (Prednisone) pills very frequently for my Asthma, I ran across some books and publications that opened my mind to try alternate remedies.

1) I started drinking Magnetized water every day as there were no side effects or interaction with my drugs for Asthma. One thing I must say Asthma patients should drink more water.

Keep the body hydrated. The benefits of drinking magnetized water are realized very slowly but it helps heart and lungs. It basically removes deposits from arteries and air passages in the lungs. Mind you, western medicine does not recognize this. Benefits of magnetized water would be another kindle book. If interested check this link but not required at all. http://www.amazon.com/dp/B007IO7DN8 or simply email me at pjan86@gmail.com for a free report on this.

By Age 60, I was completely free from Asthma. Now I cannot prove Magnetized water did it. Main stream medical practitioners will make a fun of this. I got off my inhalers and Prednisone cortisone pills which by the way affect bone density. I slowly improved my bone density with exercise, Calcium and Vitamin D.

2) I investigated Chelation Therapy. I found a certified Doctor, M.D. then in our small town in Ohio. She was certified to do the procedure of administering by I V, EDTA (Ethylene diamine tetra acetic acid) compound, approved by FDA for treating lead toxicity in the blood. I could see her clinic full of patients hooked up

to portable I V, reading books or working on their paper work. It was sight to be seen.

I decided to take two treatments a week, for six weeks. I never did consult my primary physician. I felt safe taking the treatment as a precaution to avoid heart problems in the future due to family history. I also had personal interest to see how it feels so that I can tell others my own experience. Once again I cannot recommend anything. There are several books on the subject. In this report I will cover more details.

The best part now is that at age 75+ I have no Asthma and my heart is healthy but I do take small dose of prescribed medicine for cholesterol to keep it under control. I do consume red meat, fish and drink red wine. I am currently taking additional few Chelation treatments to help clean up my arteries as a precaution. I am working with an approved doctor trained and certified by ACAM for Chelation.

1- Herbs That Help Your Heart

Caution: If you are already on blood thinners like Warfin, please visit this website and consult your doctor before using any herbs described here.

http://www.naturalhomeandgarden.com/natural-health/herbs-heart-health-13-herbal-remedies-heart-medication.aspx#ixzz28wnkwPlA

Arjuna

If we were to pick one of the best herb for maintaining healthy heart, reduce LDL, improve HDL, reduce stress, regulate blood pressure, improve liver functions, get protection against E-Coli and fight against bone cancer, we should be picking Arjuna herb. As many good things in life like air and water are almost free, but in essence priceless, this herb is very in expensive but offers great benefits.

If you are 50+ years old consider investigating this herb and start using it. Benefits with many herbs come slowly but last longer. As always do your research to avoid conflict with your prescription drugs if any. Your main stream doctor may or may not be the best judge but you can ask the manufacturer of herb and doctors who prescribe alternate medicines.

This most valuable herb comes from India from Arjuna Tree.

It is a powerful tonic for cardiac activities as prescribed by Ayurvedic practitioners. The plant grows to 60-90 feet high as an evergreen tree all over India. It has a spreading crown and drooping branches. The bark of this tree is very thick and smooth, grey or pinkish green in color.

The bark of this tree has been in use for over 2000 years to help our hearts stay healthy. This herb helps regulate blood circulation and promotes cardiac health. Its principle constituents are Arjunolic acid, ßsitosterol, Ellagic acid and Triterpenoid saponin.

Arjuna has been tested for effectiveness against nitroglycerin most commonly prescribed for increasing blood supply to the heart and it has proven to be effective regardless of duration of use. However nitroglycerin's effect is reduced with each use.

Use of Arjuna has no side effects compared to nitroglycerin based drugs causing dizziness and a rapid pulse rate and light headedness.

* Arjuna supports to reduce the effects of stress and nervousness. It helps to regulate Blood pressure and promotes healthy cardiac functioning. It has demonstrated antioxidant properties comparable to Vitamin E and is helpful as an anti-ischemic and cardio protective agent in hypertension and ischemic heart disease, especially in disturbed cardiac rhythm, angina and myocardial infarction. It has a diuretic and a general tonic effect in case of cirrhosis of liver.

Arjuna is also very effective in reducing LDL, improving HDL and reducing systolic blood pressure levels. Arjuna can help lower Cholesterol as much as 64%. People taking this herb preparation see their LDL levels plummet by an average of 25.6%.

If you have a family history of heart disease Arjuna is the herb to take as a preventive measure. One of the best and very affordable herb to protect you against atherosclerosis also known as hardening of the arteries.

Interesting enough Arjuna has powerful antibacterial properties against E.coli and bacteria causing pneumonia, bladder and kidney infections. Arjuna contains ellagic acid to fight against food poisoning caused by Salmonella gastroenteritis.

Amazing as it may sound research has shown Arjuna also is effective against cancer stopping all mutation which is the start of causing cancer to normal cells. As such Arjuna is a wonder herb and proving its worth even against growth of bone cancer.

Available in USA: Himalaya Herbal Healthcare, 10440 West Office Drive, Houston,

TX 77042. 800-869-4640 or visit www.himalayausa.com

The Himalaya Drug company is very reputable company with HQ located in Bangalore, India. Also available from Amazon.com and other suppliers on the web. We have no connection with any suppliers.

Recommended dosage: 1 capsule twice a day before meals.

Warning: Do not use if you have ailing or weak kidneys or if you are using blood thinners.

Note: If you are under a doctor's care or taking any prescription drugs, please consult your medical advisor before taking this potent herb.

If you are Pregnant, nursing or planning to become pregnant consult your health care Professional before using any herbal Products.

Garlic

Another least expensive natural herb easily available around the globe if consumed daily has proven to lower LDL and improve HDL cholesterol levels. If possible take a clove or two a day. The beneficial sulfur compound in Garlic is allicin. When a clove of garlic is either crushed, chewed or cut, this sulfur compound is instantly formed giving it that famous odor and it is also responsible for its medicinal values.

The Garlic is rich in sulfur compounds and belongs to Onion family. It has more than 200 medicinal uses dated back to ancient times. Here are some worth knowing

* Helps regulate blood sugar
* Reduces high blood pressure
* Garlic tea fights off cold and cough symptoms. Add honey for additional benefits
* It has antiseptic and anti-fungal properties
* Garlic seems to help decrease the risk of colorectal and Prostate Cancer
* It has anti-inflammatory and anti-viral properties
* Since ancient times it has been also effective against arthritis
* It seems to help avoid cataracts of the eye

* Apart from Allicin, garlic has potassium, zinc, polyphenols, vitamin B6, phosphorus and vitamin C, selenium and manganese.

All this to fight heart disease and provide protection against cancer and more.

Cayenne

Another wonder spice from India. Just be careful using a small pinch to a glass of juice, or a bowl of cooked food. If you are not used to spicy hot taste, go slow to start. Slowly increase the use of it. I personally cook with it as curry powder and sprinkle it over cooked food including my Yogurt. This very common herb stimulates the blood flow and is effective against hardening of arteries and has toning effect on the heart. It is a powerful anti-inflammatory agent and prevents formation of blood clots hence reducing the chances of stroke. Helps maintain healthy blood pressure and reduces LDL and Triglycerides. It is equally effective against acidity, ulcers and diarrhea. In addition it is effective against cold

and Flu symptoms and helps prevent Migraine.
Use it wisely.

Amazing Age Old Recipe to Open Clogged Arteries

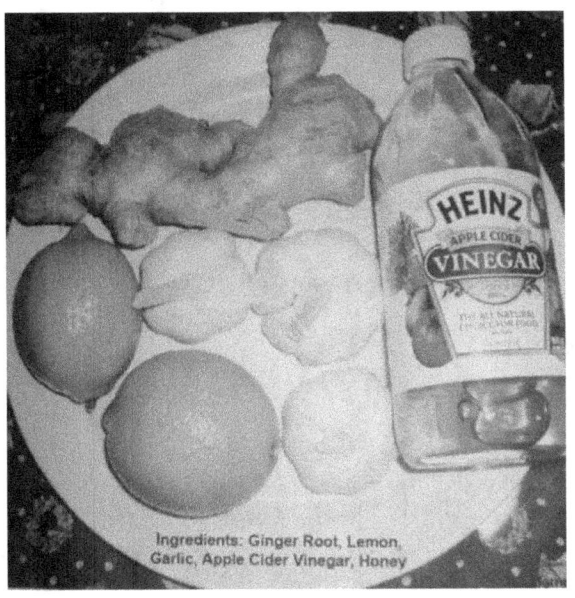

Ingredients: Ginger Root, Lemon, Garlic, Apple Cider Vinegar, Honey

Ingredients

1 cup Lemon juice
1 cup Ginger juice
1 cup Garlic juice
1 cup Apple cider vinegar

Mix all above and simmer in low heat for about 60 minutes or till solution reduces to 3 cups. Remove solution to cool, then mix 3 cups of natural honey and store it in a jar.

Drink one tablespoon daily before breakfast. Your vein's blockage will open in most cases. Enjoy your drink. It has a good taste too.

True Story: (Sent from Mufti Mohammed Kantharvi. London UK)

Have you been advised to undergo Angiography or Bypass?

Please Wait……………………..

Before you undergo Angiography or Bypass treatment, you must try with confidence the above remedy.

On the 18th April last year, I had to go to Sahiwaal (Pakistan) from the UK to attend the annual Khatme-e-Nabuwat conference. The day before I suffered acute pain at the place of my heart and thereafter, experienced discomfort which continued for quite some time. I then met in Pakistan Hazrat Moulana Bashir Ahmed Usmani Sahib, a herbalist and disclosed to him, that when the doctors performed Angiography on me, they advised bypass as they discovered 3 of my arteries were blocked and I was given a date to be operated after a month.

During this period, my herbalist prepared himself the same preparation as described above to unclog the arteries, using fresh lemon juice, ginger, garlic, vinegar and honey. As per instructions I consumed this remedy exactly for a month.

A day before my bypass operation, I arrived at the Cardiology Hospital in Lahore (Pakistan) and deposited Pak Rs. 225,000.00 towards expenses for my bypass surgery. After taking a close look at the results and my previous results, the Doctors then asked me if I had taken any medication after the previous tests were carried out.

I told them of Hakim Sahibs prescribed remedy. The panel of Doctors, surprised by the results, then informed me that according to the latest reports all 3 arteries were open and functioning normally and that surgery was not required. I was refunded my deposit and told to go home. A happy ending and what a relief!

2- Power of Pomegranate

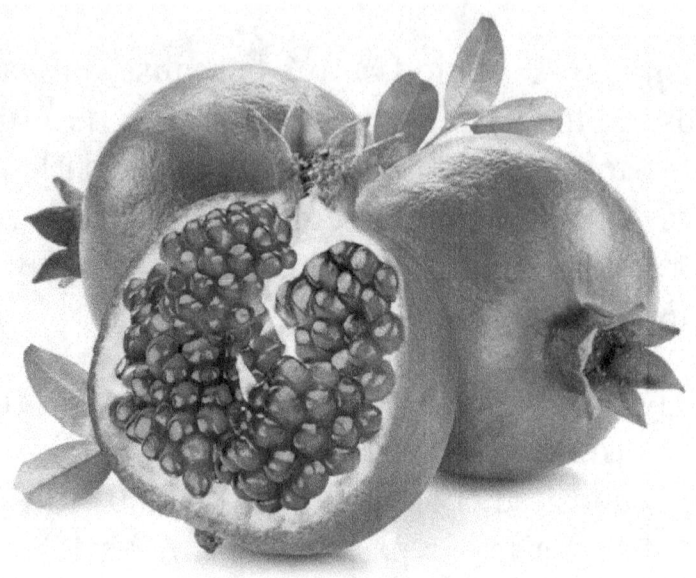

As submitted by Dr.Thahira Kukkady:

Two things are full of benefits for the human being....lukewarm water and pomegranate.

An Experiment with Dried Pomegranate Seeds

I prepared a decoction boiling a fistful of **dried seeds** in half liter (about 16 oz.) of water for 10 minutes, squeezed the seeds, strained the decoction and advised those patients suffering from painful angina to use a glass of lukewarm decoction on an empty stomach in the morning.

Amazing result was observed, the decoction of dried pomegranate seeds worked like a magic, the feelings of tightness and heaviness of chest and the pain had gone.

It encouraged me to try more experiments on all types of cardiac patients so I tried other experiments on patients who were suffering from painful angina, coronary arterial blockage, cardiac ischemia (insufficient blood flow to the heart muscle) etc., waiting for a bypass surgery. The same lukewarm decoction was used on an empty stomach in the morning. The patients experienced quick relief in all symptoms including painful condition.

In another case of coronary arterial blockage the patient started using half glass of fresh pomegranate juice every day for one year, although all symptoms were completely relieved within a week but he continued taking it for a whole year, it completely reversed the plaque build-up and unblocked his arteries to normal, the angiography report confirmed the evidence.

Thus, the decoction of dried pomegranate seeds, fresh pomegranate juice or eating a whole pomegranate on an empty stomach in the morning, proved to be a miracle cure for cardiac patients.

But, the lukewarm dried seeds decoction proved to be more effective compared to eating a whole pomegranate or fresh pomegranate juice.

A regular use of pomegranate in any of the above ways ensures a healthy cardiac life, thinning your blood, dissolving the blood clots and obstructions inside the coronary arteries, maintains an optimal blood flow, supports a healthy blood pressure, prevents and reverses atherosclerosis (thickening of the internal lining of the blood vessels). From whatever I have experienced and observed in the last several years, I can say:

"A pomegranate a day keeps the Cardiologist away."

You can try and see the wonder!!

According to Dr. Fuhrman, Juice of pomegranate is full of antioxidants more than compared to red wine, green tea, blueberries and cranberries.

Compounds known as Punicalagins are the key ingredients found only in pomegranates. These compounds help lower cholesterol and blood pressure. Further they speed up the process to remove the heart blockages.

3- Chelation Therapy, How It Works, Where To Seek Help

Chelation Therapy has been in medical use for decades to treat the patients intoxicated with heavy metals like lead, mercury, arsenic and many others.

The procedure involves use of FDA approved chelating agents like ethylene diamine tetra acetic acid (EDTA). Di mercapto succinic acid (DMSA) is another chelating agent used for the treatment of lead poisoning in children.

However chelation therapy has not been approved by FDA for anything other than removal of heavy metals. Nevertheless Alternative medicine practitioners frequently use chelation therapy for helping patients with Heart disease.

Hardening of arteries reduces the flow of blood through them thus affecting the much needed nourishment and oxygen to different parts of body. However administration of EDTA intravenously has proven time and time again effective against reversing the hardening of arteries and improving the blood flow.

The treatment is almost painless. You simply lie down or sit up hooked up to an IV drip, read your book, sip on water, or simply relax and watch TV. The process takes about an hour and a half per sitting, depending upon your dosage. I am told 3 grams is full dose (bag) and one can start with half of that (half bag). You are encouraged to take a drink of water frequently as you would make a trip or two to empty your bladder to flush out the toxins. The procedure is conducted and supervised under a qualified medical practitioner. Your doctor will normally order blood test for you before and after few treatments to check your kidney function. Also your doctor will decide the total number and the frequency of these treatments depending on your situation. So basically the chelating agent like EDTA binds with the deposits and heavy metals in your blood and thus slowly flushing them out in your urine. Hence the importance of drinking water.

Introducing Integrative Medicine

According to ACAM integrative medicine combines conventional care with alternative medicine to improve patient care. Rather than practice one type of medicine, integrative physicians will often combine therapies and treatment approaches to ensure the best results for their patients. ACAM physicians do not shun western medicine; in fact they practice western care every day. These physicians are unique in that they incorporate appropriate and proven alternative treatment options.

Introducing ACAM-American College for Advancement in Medicine

ACAM organization located in Irvine California, trains and certify all licensed healthcare providers, including M.D's, DO's, ND's, PhD's and DC's and many more in integrative medicine. Chelation Therapy is one example. They maintain a list of certified Chelation therapists around the world.

Contact ACAM in USA at 1-800-532-3688

Monday-Friday 8:00 AM - 5:00 PM Mountain Time or click on to this link:

http://acam.site-ym.com/search/custom.asp?id=1758

Click on Health Resources and select Physician+ link.

Then select from Specialties "Chelation Therapy" from drop down list. Select country, and hit continue. You should have list of doctors certified by ACAM.

(Note: In some countries you may not find any doctor).

Note: Some of these treatments may not be covered by your medical insurance.

Important Note: Readers are advised to be careful about using Oral Chelation products. Research shows that it may take a very long time, months or years in some cases to see any desired benefits. However intravenous Chelation Therapy many times is able to achieve these required benefits in days. Unfortunately IV therapy could be expensive as it may not be covered by your medical insurance. In that case Oral Chelation would be an alternate choice.

Reported Benefits of Chelation Therapy:

* Lowers Cholesterol
* Helps lower blood pressure
* Helps getting rid of cramps
* Curb the Hair loss and even grow new hair
* Reduce insulin dependence. Great for diabetics
* Improve eye sight and avoid cataracts
* Even post-surgery cataract patients will enjoy fully restored sight
* *Sharpen memory and mental functions
* look younger with less wrinkles and healthy nails
* Avoid cold feet and hands and improve physical energy
* Improved sex life
* Reduce allergies
* Improve cardiac health

* Excellent cure for Alzheimer's disease
* *Helps maintain ideal weight
* *Reduces pain from arthritis

The list goes on.

The Chelation Process

Before actual treatment is scheduled your doctor should run your necessary lab reports for blood, urine and kidney functions. Also should check your blood for metal toxicity and go over your medical history including blood pressure and blood sugar. This would help your doctor to adjust your EDTA dosage and frequency of treatments. Your doctor knows best. Just follow his/her advice. If your primary doctor has covered some of these tests very recently you should take copies of these reports to this doctor, if you can. However I warn you if you will ask your primary doctor about Chelation therapy, most probably he will not approve it. You see main stream medical practitioners do not believe in these treatments.

However when it was their own health involved these same doctors in several cases have opted for Chelation. According to

National Institute of Health, over 800,000 patients opted for Chelation therapy in the United States in a single year!

Kindly note this process is also advisable for heart patients who have already gone through the bypass as chances are the vein grafts used in bypass do get clogged again within next year or two. The chelation has been successfully used even for patients over age 90; hence age is not an issue factor normally.

The process itself is painless. It is intravenous prick with a needle to start the EDTA drip.

Though you are tied to IV equipment, mostly on wheels, you are free to move or use restroom as your arm is properly secured with tape. You can also simply sit with pillow supporting your back or lie down. You are free to move about, talk to other patients undergoing the same treatment, read a book or do your office / paper work, or watch TV or bring your kindle to read books like these. It is always a pleasant atmosphere.

Trust me I have personally taken 12 treatments in year 2000 and now at age 75, I am planning to take few more treatments soon. One of the reason I have generated this kindle publication is to let people know that I am talking from my own experience as well. As they say it is better to die healthy when you are very old than to die young and unhealthy.

Normal duration of this treatment is between 1-2 hours. You will start seeing some benefits after 4 to 5 treatments. Ten to 30 treatments are common depending upon your personal medical issues. You can also ask your doctor if you are a good candidate for a lower dosage (or half a bag) treatments saving you time and may be money.

Make sure you communicate well with your doctor, if Chelation makes you feel dizzy or uncomfortable, weak or lethargic due to low blood pressure possibly. 99% of the times I believe you will have no side effects. EDTA is a mild diuretic and if you have frequent visits to bathroom consider that as a good sign. Drink plenty of water to help flush your kidneys.

Typical costs for Chelation treatment in USA

1) Consultation with doctor and evaluation-----$200.

2) Your doctor may order blood test to make sure your kidneys and liver are fine to take Chelations.- $100+

3) First Chelation to check metal toxicity------$125.00

4) Cost of the Lab to check urine sample collected from first test --$100+

5) After receiving the Lab results, your doctor will establish number of EDTA Chelations and frequency to start with. It is normal to get Chelations twice/week for 10 weeks. Each chelations costs about $125.00.

6) My doctor charges up front and then bills my insurance who pay me directly for covered services. Since removal of toxic metals, like lead, by EDTA infusions, Intra Venus (I V) method, is approved by FDA in the United States, most of the insurance companies do cover the procedure in USA.

7) In my case here in USA, Medicare and my supplemental insurance almost covered the 90% of the cost. Most of the insurance companies also cover the Lab fees as well. Mine did.
8) However if you have a HMO plan your coverage will vary.

Note: The side benefit of EDTA Chelations is that it does help clean your arteries and improve your circulation. That is the purpose of this book to explain those benefits.

Comment: Even if you have to pay a bunch from your pocket to treat your conditions, I highly recommend you. It will be lot less than going to emergency and get treated for heart issues and lingering repeat procedures after surgery, if required.

Chelations if taken seriously will avoid heart related and several other issues as explained in this book.

Let Us Now Examine Some Actual Case Histories

These case histories are collected from several sources as described below:

Source: "Everything You Should Know About Chelation Therapy" by Dr. Morton Walker and Dr. Hitendra Shah. This is a great book to read.

1. R. H. is blind in his left eye as a result of a childhood accident. Unfortunately he goes blind on the other eye as well. His doctor told him, there is nothing that can be done for him. However after 7 Chelation sessions his vision returns and at the same distance he reads better than his doctor!

2. Stewart F. an assembly-line foreman, was at the point of losing his gangrenous big toe. However 20 Chelation treatments saved his foot.

3. Harold W. H, M.D., was genetically predisposed to die early from a heart attack (like his father and grandfather and

many other family members). He was advised to give up working as a doctor, as the stress involved aggravated his condition. After a first early heart attack, he received a classic combination of Chelation treatments and improved his diet and lifestyle. He returned to full health and was able to resume his duties.

4. John H. M.D., Clinical Professor of Surgery, has given over 16.000 Chelation infusions to his patients. He uses EDTA Chelation on himself. At the age of 70, he is still operating 15 hours a day.

5. Ophelia, 79, had a series of strokes. She was no longer able to walk alone. After more strokes she was hospitalized for the second time, then sent home, where she suffered yet another stroke, which paralyzed her so that she couldn't swallow anymore. Her children prepared for her death, but the old lady hung on to life for another three weeks. Her ankles were swollen and fluid was in the base of her lungs. She could not hear. She was

semi-comatose - slipping in and out of sleep. Then, one of her sons arrived with news about Chelation therapy. Her doctor could not promise the family anything, as their Mamma was so far gone. She received the therapy, and improved steadily. The paralysis left. She re-learned everything she had lost: eating, drinking, talking coherently, moving around first with a walker, then without. Her first Chelation course consisted of 21 infusions. Later she took 20 more, at intervals of several months between series of 5. She is now well and carrying on a productive life. Her hearing has returned, and her appetite (that she had lost) is so good the family says she eats anything put in front of her, including Italian wine and sausage!

6. D.D. head of three corporations, found himself unable to function. Not only his brain failed, also his heart and his eyes. He was lucky to find the clinic of Dr. Evers, who gave him a special diet,

exercise and Chelation therapy. After this treatment, D.D. was back to normal life.

7. A 46 year old woman from Texas, was brought to a Dr. Deiter because she was suddenly absolutely demented. She failed to recognize her husband or her grown children or her friends. A hair analysis found her to be super- saturated with mercury. After just a week of daily Chelation, she regained her senses.

8. A 58 year old attorney was legally blind from macular degeneration. School medicine had tried their standard procedures but could not halt the progress of the degenerative process. He decided to improve his diet and administer Chelation therapy. After less than 4 months he could read and even drive again.

9. C.C., a police officer, had three coronary artery blockages, one of 85%, one of 80%, and one of 75%. His cardiologist told him that he was beyond surgery - he was a goner! He decided to fight, and

arrived in Dr. Evers' hospital in a wheelchair. After 7 weeks of Chelation treatment he went back to his job, which included picking up 200-pound drunks off the street.

10.   Dr. Leon Anderson, doctor of osteopathy, had a Parkinson's type of tremor in his right hand. He took 30 chelation infusions, but the tremor already responded after the 5th. His health was restored and he could continue to work as a doctor.

11.   Nick J. was hit by a series of unusual problems following a car accident. He suffered intense chest pains, and spells of unconsciousness. Within two years, he received 117 Chelations, his symptoms cleared up and the blackouts disappeared.

12.   Warren M. Levin, M.D., used Chelation therapy on his patients but also on himself, as a prevention, having lost his father at the age of 56, without having any pressing need of his own. He noticed

a very remarkable improvement in his memory functions.

13.   Dr. R. H. a chiropractor, whose gangrenous diabetic legs were saved from amputation by only 15 Chelation infusions.

14.   Paul M. a car assembly supervisor and chain smoker, had a whole list of complaints based on bad blood circulation. Hypertension, chest pain and muscle cramps were among them. 20 Chelation sessions gave him his health back. The blood pressure returned to normal after the 4th.

15.   Alfred was told by a surgeon that he was in dire danger of death. He needed open heart surgery to correct his angina, but the mortality risk for him would be 50%. Aubrey agreed to the operation, but was not a fit enough candidate, was refused the operation and sent home to die. After receiving a course of Chelation therapy, he was again fit enough to walk four miles daily before breakfast. A new

test found his heart good and his lungs clear, he was no longer a cardiac patient. But Medicare, his health care organization, refused to pay his bill in the amount of $364. The operation together with the hospital bill, amounting to $ 75,000, would have been paid, but as the treatment that cured him was "experimental and not tested" and "not considered the usual and customary treatment", he had to pay for it out of his own pocket.

16.   Lester I, doctor of osteopathy, had an early warning and Chelation recommendation by a colleague, which he ignored. Only after his near-fatal heart attack 5 months later, where he needed electric shocks to bring his enlarged heart back to life, did he start the first 30 chelation infusions. He returned to full health.

Source: Forty Something Forever-A consumer's guide to CHELATION THERAPY and other Heart-Savers. Harold & Arline Brecher.

1. 61 year old patient was suffering from peripheral vision due to diabetic retinopathy and could not drive. Dr. Michael Schachter (New York) started him on Chelation therapy. After just four treatments there was 50% improvement in his vision. His ophthalmologist was astounded! This patient almost legally blind now could drive his car again.

2. This 82 year old lady could no longer read, knit or watch TV and suffered great depression and anger due to her limitations. She started Chelation treatments out of desperation. After her fifth treatment she happen to glance outside her bedroom window and noticed her neighbor's dog running across her front lawn. Eureka! She screamed with joy and thanked God and ran outside to see the flowers, blue sky and started

shouting with joy to a pleasant surprise of her neighbors!

3. 86 year old man in Texas, could not recognize his wife any more after 61 years of marriage. Dr. Fox cured him with Chelation treatments and this man was normal to celebrate his diamond wedding anniversary.

4. This 68 year old lady almost had lost her mind. She could not remember things. She would go upstairs to get something and forget the reason. She would go to mailbox and open the letter just put there for mailing. Family decided to seek legal advice to declare her incompetent. They were afraid she might hurt herself. Then a neighbor suggested to try Chelation. For next three months with this treatment she gradually started to come out of her condition till she recovered fully with her memory intact and became the loving person she was!

5. James had a terrible memory loss and even could not remember his own name.

After just six Chelation treatments his mental faculties were fully restored. He began giving lectures about Chelation benefits to his fellow retirement village residents.

6. 1980 study undertaken by Swiss scientists from institution of radiation therapy and nuclear medicine at the University of Zurich comes to a dramatic conclusion: Chelation with EDTA cuts the incidence of Cancer by 90%.

My Personal Story

Recently I took 6 additional EDTA Chelation treatments. One a week. I had amazing positive results. I was on 50 mg of Losartan for B.P. and 20 mg of Lipitor for my Cholesterol before the treatment.

After the six treatments I quit my BP medications and it has been two months now my BP is normal. I reduced my Lipitor to 10 mg per day. My Lipid profile was excellent after the Chelation. My total Cholesterol dropped from 187 to 140 and Triglycerides dropped from 199 to 119 and LDL bad cholesterol dropped from 92 to 72.

I am amazed I am off the BP prescription. My primary doctor does not know about chelations I took. However he was very happy with my lipid Profile and BP.

P.S. You may get a laugh at what I am about to tell you. However there is more truth to this than you may know. I read somewhere monkeys do not have heart problems. The secret is practice walking on your four like the little kids do before they learn to balance on their feet and learn to walk.

So walk or crawl on floor inside your house over the carpet areas, including going up the stairs few times a day as an adult on your two feet and two hands. At first you may be out of breath if you are an older person but stay with it and slowly practice it daily. Apart from getting a laugh, you will benefit.

4- Magnetized Water, History, How To Make It At Home

Some decades ago, Russian scientists faced a major industrial problem. When **water flows through pipelines of a Boiler or an Engine machinery, some deposits from the water cling to the walls of the pipes**. Over time, the passage becomes narrower and the delivery of water to the machinery is reduced. The efficiency, fuel consumption and mechanical strength of the machine is therefore reduced.

While researching on this problem, scientists noticed that such **undesirable deposits did not occur in those pipes with water that was magnetized**. This started the use of magnetized water for industrial use in countries where water source is less than desirable.

One theory is when water passes through a magnetic field, the Hydrogen ion and dissolved minerals in the water get charged. The charge causes separation of minerals from water. That makes the water soft and there is improvement in taste.

Scientists became highly interested in studying magnetism. Water is a transparent fluid that has no color, odor, shape or taste of its own. It takes the shape of its container and the color, odor and taste of other things mixed with it. It is a near-universal solvent. It has the property of being able to assimilate the properties of other things. Researchers found when a permanent magnet is kept in contact with water for a considerable time; the water gets magnetically charged and acquires magnetic properties. Such magnetized water has its effect even on the human body when taken internally and regularly for a considerable period.

Use of Magnets in Healing

Ancient people have used magnetized water also without understanding its mechanism of action. Streams flowing over natural magnets in the shape of stones and boulders became magnetized and their water, when consumed by the people of that age, provided miraculous cures and energy.

In India, the Magneto therapy is an ancient therapy. Literature indicates the use of magnets to stop bleeding thousands of years ago.

In recent decades, there has been a resurgence in the use of magnets in healing of a variety of ailments, primarily in pain control of **chronic degenerative diseases such as arthritis**.

Researchers at the Medical University of South Carolina recently reported that cleaning the teeth with water from a magnetized irrigator can reduce calculus formation by over 60 per cent and improve overall gum health.

How Magnets Work

Magnets have two poles, North and South. It is based on Nature's law. Every cell in the human body can be viewed as a small magnetic unit. This property is present in all organs. Each cell produces its own magnetic field. Any disturbance in this magnetic field indicates a disorder. This equilibrium can be restored with the help of magnets, according to many researchers.

Technically, magnetism works because it increases the **speed of sedimentation** of suspended particles in water (and other liquids) and **enhances conductivity** as well as the process of ionization or dissociation of atoms and molecules into electrically charged particles. (New Scientist, June 1992.)

Physics shows that chemicals change weight, under the influence of magnetic fields; so does water. More hydroxyl (OH-) ions are created to form calcium bicarbonate and other alkaline molecules. It is these molecules that help **reduce acidity**.

Normal tap water has a pH level of about 7, whereas magnetized water can reach 7.8 pH after exposure to a 7000 gauss strength magnet for a long period of time. Diseased cells do not survive well in an alkaline environment.

Magnets also affect the bonding angle between the hydrogen and the oxygen atom in the water molecule. Magnetized water causes the hydrogen-oxygen bond angle within the water molecule to be reduced from 104 to 103 degrees. **This in turn causes the water molecule to cluster together in groups of 6-7 rather than 10-12. The smaller cluster leads**

to better absorption of water across cell walls.

There have been numerous reports, of people being cured of many chronic degenerative disease such as renal stones and arthritis, with drinking magnetized water daily.

Human Applications

Experience has shown that magnetized water contributes and helps in the treatment of many diseases. It is especially beneficial in treating **digestive, nervous, urinary disorders, and chronic degenerative diseases**. Some researchers have pointed out the apparent differences between water exposed to the north versus the South Pole.

The effects of the North Pole (negative) and South Pole (positive) magnetism are quite different. North polarity stabilizes, calms and sedates and also reduces pain, infection and inflammation. South polarity, on the other hand, is acid producing, enervating, biologically disorganizing and may accelerate bacteria growth. Magnets with a South polarity should only be used under the care of a trained practitioner if at all.

The degree of magnetization of liquids depends on three things:

1. The quantity of liquid being magnetized.
2. The power of the magnet used for the purpose.
3. The duration of the contact of the liquid container with the magnet.

Although we can measure the power of a magnet, we have no method of measuring the degree of magnetization of liquid. In the absence of any definite measure, only experience can guide us.

A simple way to magnetize water is to keep a bottle of water on top of strong encased disc magnet (North Pole) of about 3000 gauss strength, normally for twelve to twenty-four hours. In stationary magnetization it is important to ensure that only negatively polarized water (North Pole) or mixed negative and positive water (South Pole) is used.

A simpler and more modern way is to have water pass through magnetic discs of up to 10,000 gausses momentarily in order to achieve a similar effect. Such Magnets can be installed permanently under the sink or at cold water inlet at the service entrance in the house. Visit my website www.Healingwithmagnets.org and scroll down on the home page to see under the sink water magnet. I use this on inlet pipe feeding our dish washer to improve quality of rinse and reducing spots on glassware.

Health Benefits

The reported health benefits of magnetized water are many, including:

Acidity and Other Digestive Disorders: Magnetized water reduces excess acidity and bile in the digestive system. It helps to regulate the movement of the bowels expelling all accumulations of poisonous matter.

Kidney Stones: The use of magnetic water in urinary and kidney disorders has been documented. In scientific studies, magnetic water has been prescribed to persons suffering from renal calculus. An adult suffering from renal stone is advised to drink one-liter of magnetized water per day, while in case of children it is 500ml per day. Results have been very encouraging. I have testimonials from my customers who have benefited.

Low Blood Pressure and Nervous System: Magnetized water is also very beneficial for nervous disorders and treatment of blood pressure, especially low blood pressure. It gives a soothing and slightly sedative effect to the nerves, **aids in clearing clogged arteries**, and normalizes the circulatory system. Please be advised benefits will be noticeable after a long and consistent use of M-water. However the results will also be long lasting. I advise keep drinking this water every day as you would anyway.

Asthma/Bronchitis: Magnetized water is effective in the treatment of asthma, bronchitis, colds, coughs and certain types of fevers. Once again benefits come slowly and surely. I cured my Asthma of 20+ years. However I still drink M-water every day.

Watch my You Tube video

http://www.youtube.com/watch?feature=player
_embedded&v=7GLvxync89E#t=6s

Healing of Wounds: Magnetized water has been used as an external aid for washing swollen and sore eyes, wounds, eczema spots, etc. for quicker healing. In all types of eye infections, north pole magnetized water has healing and anti-biotic type properties.

Magnetized water is softer than tap water so magnetization can result in significant savings in detergent and soap use. It also helps prevent deposits on cutlery and glasses washed in a dish washer and can even make hair shinier.

Conclusion:

The use of magnetized water in the treatment of chronic diseases is still in the **infancy stage of investigation**. Magnetism is widely used in medical diagnostics, including Magnetic Resonance Scanning (MRI) devices for detection of a variety of internal organ dysfunction, including cancer.

There is very little doubt that our cells react like a tiny magnet throughout the body's universe. Disturbance of this balance may bring on dysfunction of the body that current tests and investigative tools are simply not sensitive enough to measure.

It will be decades before the science of magnetized water is fully understood. Those in mainstream medicine may discount magnetized water as "quackery". Those in the forefront of magnetic research paint a different story. If one understands and accepts that each of our cells possess a small magnetic field, as many research studies are now supporting, the **logical conclusion that magnetic water has the ability to affect our cells must be taken seriously**.

In the end, the truth probably lies somewhere in between - magnetized water is not a magic panacea or cure-all. It is also not a total quackery and most likely will turn out to be a health-enhancing medium.

It enhances our health in at least two ways.

Magnetized water increases the alkalinity of water. An alkaline pH balances the biological terrain as our body is bathed in a pro-cancer acid environment from a modern day meat heavy diet and pollution.

Magnetized water also leads to a reduction in the cluster size of water molecules, leading to better absorption of water into the cell.

SUMMARY

Benefits of Magnetized Water:

Magnetic Water promotes more Alkaline pH in the body.

Promotes healing of wounds and burns.

Magnetic water has therapeutic effect on digestive, nervous and urinary system.

Magnetic water revitalizes the body.

It has been reported to help regulate heart functions and clear clogged arteries.

It has been beneficial for Kidney ailments, gout and premature aging.

Magnetized water infuses energy into the body, controls bacteria and stimulates brain function.

It is beneficial in Asthma.

Fluids other than water, including wine can also be magnetized.

Disclaimer: Above information should not be taken as medical advice. It is simply a collection of information from various sources. Please consult your Medical Doctor for further advice. We do not make or imply any medical claims for any procedure or products.

This Is What I Follow

Place a water bottle on top of the magnet North (Blue side) all the time. Then drink from this bottle. Every time I drink, as much I want, I put the bottle back on the magnet. So bottle stays on the magnet all the time. I Refill or replace the bottle when empty and place it back on the magnet. I use disposable 16 oz. plastic bottles.

Drink all the water you can and enjoy the benefits. The benefits will come slowly but surely.

PLEASE READ THIS FIRST BEFORE USING MAGNETS...

Despite the safety of magnets, there are some contraindications to be aware of. First, do not use magnets during pregnancy, on those who have a history of epilepsy, those wearing a pacemaker or other metal implants that might be dislodged by exposure to magnets. Strong magnets should be used with care on small infants and children, on the eyes, the brain or over the heart.

Summary of Precautions in the Handling and Use of Magnets

Remove battery powered wristwatches and any other magnetic objects whose field can be altered by the presence of an externally applied magnet.

Avoid dropping, banging or heating magnets above 700 degrees Fahrenheit as this may dissipate their strength.

Be careful in handling large heavy magnets as one can injure a body part if they were to suddenly slam together and pinch your fingers or hand. Best way to separate two stuck magnets isto slide them apart rather than try and pull them apart.

If possible, do not allow different sized magnets to remain together.

Keep magnets away from homeopathic remedies, computer hard drives, recording tape, credit cards, and videos to prevent them being damaged or erased.

5- Heart Health and Use of Water

Correct time to drink water... Very Important. From A Cardiac Specialist!

Drinking water at a certain time maximizes its effectiveness on the body:

2 glasses of water after waking up - helps activate internal organs

1 glass of water 30 minutes before a meal - helps digestion

1 glass of water before taking a bath - helps lower blood pressure

1 glass of water before going to bed - avoids stroke or heart attack

Drinking water at bed time will also help prevent night time leg cramps. Your leg muscles are seeking hydration when they cramp and wake you up with a Charlie's Horse.

If you take an aspirin or a baby aspirin once a day, take it at night.

The reason: Aspirin has a 24-hour "half-life"; therefore, if most heart attacks happen in the wee hours of the morning, the Aspirin would be strongest in your system.

6- Nitric Oxide and How It Can Help Circulation

It may be of surprise to you that many health problems such as blood pressure, cholesterol, blood sugar, stiff arteries, diminished memory, poor vision... even depleted sex drive could be caused by poor circulation.

Once your circulation is fine, oxygen and nutrient-rich blood will get to every corner of your body helping to:

Support a healthy heart

Increase stamina and energy levels

Enhance memory and concentration

Promote healthy vision and hearing

Promote healthy cholesterol

Support healthy blood sugar levels

Enhance sexual performance

With good and healthy circulation, oxygen and nutrient rich blood can reach

The tiny capillaries in your eyes so your vision stays sharp.

The deepest parts of your brain for stronger memory and clear focus.

Every organ and tissue cell for greater energy and stamina.

The sexual organs for more enjoyable sex.

In addition you will be able to get rid of your toxins.

All You Need Is This Miracle Supplement!

Taking this supplement is like opening the floodgates and flooding your body with health, energy and vitality. It will make you feel years younger and you will be able to enjoy each day with renewed vigor.

Opens arteries. Improves blood flow.
Supports healthy blood pressure.

Boosts energy. Revs up sexual
performance... and so much more.

When the researcher, Louis Ignarro, M.D., discovered what this molecule does for us, he was awarded the Nobel Prize in Medicine in 1998.

The Nobel-Prize Winning "Miracle
Molecule" You've Never Heard Of!

This miracle molecule is known as *Nitric Oxide (NO)*. Please don't confuse this with "nitrous oxide", the laughing gas the dentist gives you. It's quite different. Nitric Oxide is a very simple molecule found naturally in your body. It has only two atoms—one atom of nitrogen and one atom of oxygen. Nitric Oxide is a molecule produced in your arteries, in the linings of your blood vessels, known as the endothelium (en doe-thee-le-um).

So when Nitric Oxide is produced at peak levels, your circulation immediately improves. Blood surges through your body. With good circulation, more oxygen and nutrients can now be delivered directly to all your cells keeping them healthy and functioning properly.

And with healthy circulation, your blood pressure naturally lowers, your heart pumps stronger, your brain thinks clearly, your vision improves, your hearing gets better, your energy levels soar and last but not least, even your sex life improves.

Almost 120,000 studies show that Nitric Oxide is very effective in fighting against numerous health concerns, and even reversing them. That's because Nitric Oxide boosts oxygen-rich circulation throughout your entire body. From the tiny capillaries in your eyes, to the deepest parts of your brain, to the tips of your toes and fingers, Nitric Oxide is relaxing blood vessels and making sure your blood gets where it needs to be.

As a result it:

Promotes healthy, clear arteries and veins

Supports a healthy heart

Increases energy levels

Increases stamina

Enhances memory and concentration

Promotes healthy vision

Promotes healthy cholesterol

Supports healthy blood sugar levels

Here is the summary of recommended supplements from Nobel Laureate Dr. Louis J. Ignarro for improving your Nitric Oxide levels. Please do check with your physician before using this or any other supplements. Also your doctor will check your current nitric oxide level. It is a quick check using previously treated paper strip.

L-arginine--------4000-6000 mg per day

L-citrulline ------200-1000 mg per day

Vitamin C -------500 mg/ day

Vitamin E -------200 IU / day

Folic Acid--------400-800 mcg /day

Alpha Lipoic acid--10 mg /day

These supplements can be taken with or without food any time of the day.

(Please refer to Dr. Ignarro's book "NO More Heart Disease" for full explanation)

7- Lack of Sleep Can Affect Your Heart Health

Research in England shows that a common habit of busy people hurts heart health and even compromises the ability to breathe correctly.

The problem starts when your busy schedule makes you cut back on sleep. Scientists at the University of Birmingham in the United Kingdom have found that if you sleep only about four hours a night, your blood vessels stop functioning properly and your breathing control malfunctions.

"If acute sleep loss occurs repetitively over a long period of time, then vascular health could be compromised (even) further and eventually mediate the development of cardiovascular disease," explains researcher Keith Pugh.

The scientists also believe that the loss of breathing control that they discovered could contribute to sleep apnea, another risk factor for heart disease.

Cutting Back on Sleep Harms Blood Vessel Function and Breathing Control:

Research has shown a link between sleep deprivation and cardiovascular disease.

The researchers have worked with eight healthy adult volunteers between the ages of 20 to 35 to date. For the first two nights of the study, the researchers had these volunteers sleep a normal night of eight hours. Then, rather than restrict their sleep completely, the researchers instead had them sleep only four hours during each of three consecutive nights.

Each of these volunteers underwent tests to see how well their blood vessels accommodate an increase in blood flow, a test of healthy blood vessel, or vascular function. Following the first two nights of restricted sleep, the researchers found a significant reduction in vascular function compared to following the nights of normal sleep. However, after the third night of sleep restriction, vascular function returned to baseline, possibly an adaptive response to acute sleep loss, study leader Pugh explains

In other tests, the researchers exposed subjects to moderately high levels of carbon dioxide, which normally increases the depth and rate of breathing. However, breathing control was substantially reduced after the volunteers lost sleep.

The researchers later had these volunteers sleep 10 hours a night for five nights. After completing the same tests, results showed that vascular function and breathing control had improved.

"If acute sleep loss occurs repetitively over a long period of time, then vascular health could be compromised further and eventually mediate the development of cardiovascular disease,"

Similarly, the loss of breathing control that the researchers observed could play a role in the development of sleep apnea, which has also been linked with cardiovascular disease.

So restricting sleep harms vascular function and breathing control.

8- Let Us Toast To Our Healthy Heart

Wine usually gets the heart-healthy accolades—and it should. But this other age-old drink has health benefits of its own. And they're not minor effects.

In a study published in the journal of *Nutrition*, researchers at Harokopio University in Athens found this other age old drink also improves blood flow and heart function in just two hours.

Non-smoking men who drank 400 mL—a little less than a pint—of this drink reduced their aortic stiffness. Their arteries became more flexible.

In fact, this drink improves blood-vessel function more than 50 percent…

This other drink **beer** also has several heart-helping flavonoid compounds. In just two hours, it relaxes your arteries and reduces inflammation.

Beer reduces cholesterol and increases antioxidants. It changes your blood chemistry to reduce your heart attack risk.

It also reduces levels of fibrinogen, a clot-producing protein. Beer makes the clotting protein less active and improves blood flow.

Keep your consumption to one or two drinks a day to reap the benefits without the risks. Drinking more than that negates the health benefits and will actually damage your heart.

While wine enjoys the heart-healthy spotlight, beer drinkers can rejoice too. Beer is lower in alcohol content but has just as many nutritional benefits of wine. All types of beer produce positive results. So raise a pint and let us toast to your health.

9- Amazing five Tibetan Rites

The 5 Ancient Tibetan Rites are an ancient and potent set of practices which were formulated over 2500 years ago, and are mostly practiced by Tibetan monks. They work mainly on our 7 key chakras and endocrine system thus slowing down the ageing process, reset our body to optimum functioning and fill us with a dynamic, youthful energy.

Please study the following You Tube videos placed here for you to save you time.

Additional information is available on the web.

Rite 1 - Slows Ageing, Increases Energy
http://yupurl.com/iff483
Rite 2 - Induces Vitality, Strength
http://yupurl.com/2alri5
Rite 3 - Joyfulness, Flexibility
http://yupurl.com/gtglj1
Rite 4 - Clarity, Development
http://yupurl.com/32obfu
Rite 5 - Body Toning, Tranquility
http://yupurl.com/qq6ac2
Caution For Young and Old

Start slowly just 3 to 5 times each exercise. Also do only stretches as far as you can without discomfort. You can hurt yourself

otherwise. If you like more FREE details click here:
http://www.ask.com/wiki/Five_Tibetan_Rites

Good luck.

10- Latest Medical Tests That Can Help You

Corus CAD:

What it does: Evaluates your risk for narrowing or blockage in your coronary arteries.

Why it's important: "To my knowledge, this is the only test that can tell you what's going on in your arteries at the cellular and molecular level," says physician Alan Grossman, medical director of the Nuclear Cardiology and Echocardiography Laboratories at the Heart and Vascular Center of Arizona, which this year introduced the Corus CAD test. "Using this test, we've found people with severe multi vessel coronary artery disease whom we would not have considered at high risk otherwise."

How it works: A small sample of your blood is sent to the laboratory of the test's maker, where it's screened for the presence of 23 genes that have been found to be associated with narrowing or blocked arteries.

Cost: $1,195

Covered by insurance? Some insurance companies cover this test, but many don't yet. However, the company that makes the test is committed to helping people get coverage, and it provides a patient advocate to help you through the process. And with *Time* magazine having picked Corus CAD as one of the top-ten medical breakthroughs of 2010, wider adoption and coverage are sure to come quickly.

Who should get it: The most definitive risk factor for a coronary artery blockage is chest pain, particularly chest pain or discomfort that comes on or increases when you exercise. Other risk factors: a family history of heart disease or heart attack.

The company that makes the test, CardioDX, currently offers the test in nine states: Kentucky, Maryland, Illinois, Washington, Wisconsin, Minnesota, North Carolina, Texas, and Arizona. If you don't live in one of these states, call the company for your state.

High-Sensitivity C-Reactive Protein Test:

What it does: Measures even very low blood levels of C-reactive protein (CRP), which is produced by the liver in response to inflammation. CRP is an indicator for cardiovascular disease -- among other conditions -- because chronic inflammation damages the interior of artery walls. Because hs-CRP, also called ultra-sensitive CRP or cardio CRP, is sensitive enough to detect lower concentrations of the protein, it can detect inflammation in a healthy person, indicating the early onset of cardiovascular disease.

Why it's important: This is the first new general screening test for heart disease to be recommended by the American Heart Association in 20 years. The reason: The hs-CRP takes the traditional heart checkup a step further, more accurately predicting who's at risk for heart attack, stroke, and diabetes. People whose hs-CRP results are in the high end of the normal range have 1.5 to 4 times the risk of having a heart attack than those whose hs-CRP values are at the low end of the normal range. In addition, recent studies demonstrated an association between elevated CRP levels and colon cancer.

How it works: The hs-CRP is a blood test used in concert with other tests, such as a blood pressure check and a lipid profile to check cholesterol and triglyceride levels.

Cost: $40-$70

Covered by insurance? If your doctor recommends the hs-CRP test because you have a family history of heart disease or other risk factors, most insurers, including Medicare, will cover it.

Who should get it: Currently the hs-CRP test is recommended for anyone considered to be at moderate or intermediate risk of developing cardiovascular disease in the next ten years. While hs-CRP isn't yet considered a screening tool for the general population, an important recent study called the JUPITER study found that hs-CRP predicted heart disease even in people with no risk factors, and some experts now believe everyone in their late 50s and older should have it, even if they have minimal risk factors. The test is simple and inexpensive, and your doctor can order it based on his or her recommendation. So discuss your concerns with your doctor, mention any relatives who had an early heart attack, and you should be covered.

Unfortunately, certain conditions such as arthritis, autoimmune conditions, and chronic infection also cause inflammatory response, so if you have one of these conditions, the hs-CRP test can't be used.

Genetic Analysis:

What it does: Tests you for approximately a hundred traits, providing a genetic blueprint known as a comprehensive genotype that predicts your risk of developing a variety of conditions and diseases. Genotyping also offers information on how you respond to certain key medications such as blood thinners, and it lets you know if you're a carrier for certain genetic traits.

Why it's important: Based on the genetic information you receive, you could find out if you're at risk for certain cancers,

Alzheimer's, macular degeneration, and other conditions. Knowing what may lie in your future makes you more alert for warning signs. In the case of lung cancer, diabetes, and other conditions strongly affected by lifestyle, finding out you're at risk might increase your motivation to make important changes, such as losing weight or quit smoking -- or to take specific tests to detect a condition early enough to treat it. In this case, knowledge really is power: Knowing you're at risk empowers you to take steps to protect yourself.

How it works: Personalized genotyping is done by saliva testing. Your saliva sample is collected in a tube and shipped off to a sophisticated genetic testing laboratory that analyzes your DNA. The results are ready in two to three weeks, at which point you're given access to a comprehensive report and interactive genetic counseling via a secure online account. The testing kits are provided by private companies, which include 23andme, Navigenics, and Pathway Genomics; each company then provides its own ongoing health management service.

Cost: Varies, depending on the company and the extent of the services provided. You can pay for the initial testing only, then be billed for regular monthly reports and genetic counseling; or you can pay upfront for the comprehensive service. Range is $99 plus a $5-per-month subscription access fee with a 12-month commitment, or $399-$499 for full-service access.

Covered by insurance? Insurance doesn't cover this type of comprehensive genetic analysis. However, if you have a health savings account or a flexible spending account for healthcare, you'll likely be able to use those dollars to purchase a genotyping service and submit it for reimbursement. Check with the administrator or benefits specialist to find out.

Who should get it: Anyone concerned about their genetic risk for health conditions such as cancer, macular degeneration, **heart disease**, and diabetes, particularly those already at risk due to family history or from other risk factors. If you smoke, for example, knowing your genetic risk of lung, breast, and colorectal cancer could be extremely useful. And if you carry a lot of extra weight, you might want genetic information to better evaluate your risk of diabetes and **heart disease.**

This test may or may not apply to you. I thought you should know about it.

Early CDT-Lung Test for Lung Cancer

What it does: Measures auto antibodies the immune system produces in response to lung cancer proteins, known as antigens. These auto antibodies show up early in the cancer process, which gives this test the advantage of being able to detect lung cancer before symptoms appear.

Why it's important: With an accuracy of greater than 90 percent, this brand-new test is a significant tool for assessing lung cancer risk at an early stage, says pulmonologist Keith Kelly of Paducah, Kentucky, who offers the test to his patients. Lung cancer kills more than 160,000 people a year in the U.S. -- and the reason it's so deadly is that it's rarely caught early, when tumors are operable. Currently lung cancer still has only a 16 percent five-year survival rate. "With this test as a supplement to CT scan, we can diagnose people earlier and, hopefully, finally begin to improve the survival rate," says Kelly.

How it works: A sample of your blood is sent to a laboratory, and results are sent to your doctor about a week later. A positive result means the test detected signs your immune system's been activated in response to the presence of cancer cells. In that case, your doctor will arrange for you to have an imaging scan to search for the presence of tumors. A negative test can't guarantee that you're cancer free, but it does mean your body isn't reacting visibly to the presence of protein-producing tumors.

Cost: $475

Covered by insurance? The CDT-lung cancer test is now covered by the majority of major medical insurers and is also covered by Medicare Part B. The testing company will bill your insurance provider for you.

Who should get it: Long-term smokers and former smokers are at high risk for lung cancer and qualify for this test. Exposure to radon, asbestos, or significant secondhand smoke also puts you in the high-risk category. Oncimmune, the test maker, hopes to have a breast cancer blood test based on the same science available within the next year.

Hope some of you reading this will benefit or help someone who could.

All the best.

Note: Cost for these tests may be lower by the time you read this.

Bonus Section

EAT YOUR WAY
TO
SUPER HEALTH

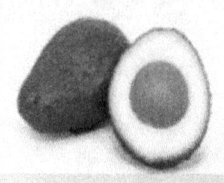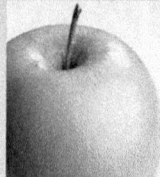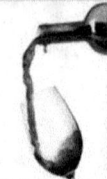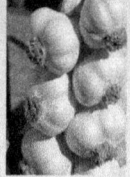

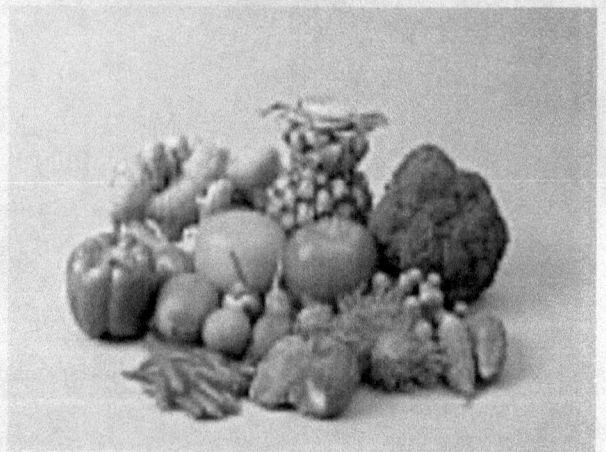

Prem Chhatwani

This brief report is a meant to be a great
ready reference
For people on the go
And
Those who are health minded individuals.
Just read which super foods presented here
Interest you most
And
Get to know them a bit better.
All the Super foods are presented
In Alphabetical order
And
Where possible
I have included additional links
For more information
And
Recipes.
Hope you will take time to explore this
report and benefit from this. Just one idea
that may benefit you directly is well worth
the effort.

Table of Contents

Chapter 1- Apples, Apricots, Artichokes and Avocados

Apples:
*Prevents Constipation (make sure you eat the skin)
One large apple has 5.7 grams of fiber which is 30% of daily requirements.
*Blocks Diarrhea
*Only 47 calories in an average size apple
* Keeps your heart healthy
*Improves Lung capacity
* Prevents type II diabetes
Apple a day does help keep the doctor away!
Apricots:
*Combats Cancer
*Controls blood Pressure
*Improves eyesight
*Slows aging process
* Shields against Alzheimer's
Artichokes:
*Improves digestion
*Lowers cholesterol
*Heart healthy
*Controls blood sugar
*Guards against liver disease

Avocados:
* The monounsaturated fat in Avocados is oleic acid, which helps lower cholesterol.
*Rich in magnesium is healthy for bones, cardiac functions and blood pressure
*Rich in Potassium which helps regulate blood pressure
*Rich in folate reduces risk for heart disease and stroke
*Rich in beta-sit sterol appears to inhibit excessive cell division preventing cancer-cell growth
* It is a powerful nutrient booster helping body to absorb nutrients from food
*Battles diabetes
*Makes your skin smooth

Chapter 2- Blueberries, Bananas, Beets, Beans and Broccoli

Blueberries:

This tiny super food is very rich antioxidant and is rich in Phytonutrients. It combats Cancer, improves your memory, and helps maintain your blood sugar. The Phytonutrients help our body cells effectively communicate with each other and help prevent growth of cancer. It is important to note that we have excellent communication between body cells to avoid degenerative brain diseases like dementia and Alzheimer's diseases. Blueberries seem to slow down and even reverse degenerative diseases.

Consume 1 to 2 cups of this healthy super food daily to avoid degenerative brain diseases and get ample vitamin E and vitamin c in addition.

New research has shown that the ellagic acid a Phytonutrient present in blueberries is responsible for cancer prevention. This ellagic acid is more so located in the seeds of these berries. The further research indicates that people who consume ellagic acid are three times less likely to develop cancer in comparison to those who do not consume foods rich in ellagic acid.

So make sure you include black and red raspberries and blueberries to your daily diet.

Bananas:

Banana really is a natural remedy for many ills. When you compare it to an apple, it has four times the protein, twice the carbohydrate, three times the phosphorus, five times the vitamin A and iron, and twice the other vitamins and minerals. It is also rich in potassium and is one of the best value foods around so maybe it's time to change that well-known phrase so that we say, 'A banana a day keeps the doctor away! Bananas contain three natural sugars - sucrose, fructose and glucose combined with fiber. A banana gives an instant, sustained and substantial boost of energy. Research has proven that just two bananas provide enough energy for a strenuous 90-minute workout. No wonder the banana is the number one fruit with the world's leading athletes. But energy isn't the only way a banana can help us keep fit. It can also help overcome or prevent a substantial number of illnesses and conditions, making it a must to add to our daily diet.

Depression: According to a recent survey undertaken by MIND amongst people suffering from depression, many felt much better after eating a banana. This is because bananas contain tryptophan, a type of protein that the body converts into serotonin, known to make you relax, improve your mood and generally make you feel happier.

PMS: Forget the pills - eat a banana. The vitamin B6 it contains regulates blood glucose levels, which can affect your mood.

Anemia: High in iron, bananas can stimulate the production of hemoglobin in the blood and so helps in cases of anemia.

Blood Pressure: This unique tropical fruit is extremely high in potassium yet low in salt, making it perfect to beat blood pressure. So much so, the US Food and Drug Administration has just allowed the banana industry to make official claims for the fruit's ability to reduce the risk of blood pressure and stroke.

Brain Power: 200 students at a Twickenham (Middlesex) school (England) were helped through their exams this year by eating bananas at breakfast, break, and lunch in a bid to boost their brain power. Research has shown that the potassium-packed fruit can assist learning by making pupils more alert.

Constipation: High in fiber, including bananas in the diet can help restore normal bowel action, helping to overcome the problem without resorting to laxatives.

Hangovers: One of the quickest ways of curing a hangover is to make a banana milkshake, sweetened with honey. The banana calms the stomach and, with the help of the honey, builds up depleted blood sugar levels, while the milk soothes and re-hydrates your system.

Heartburn: Bananas have a natural antacid effect in the body, so if you suffer from heartburn, try eating a banana for soothing relief.

Morning Sickness: Snacking on bananas between meals helps to keep blood sugar levels up and avoid morning sickness.

Mosquito bites: Before reaching for the insect bite cream, try rubbing the affected area with the inside of a banana skin. Many people find it amazingly successful at reducing swelling and irritation.

Nerves: Bananas are high in B vitamins that help calm the nervous system.

Overweight and at work? Studies at the Institute of Psychology in Austria found pressure at work leads to gorging on comfort food like chocolate and chips. Looking at 5,000 hospital patients, researchers found the most obese were more likely to be in high-pressure jobs. The report concluded that, to avoid panic-induced food cravings, we need to control our blood sugar levels by snacking on high carbohydrate foods every two hours to keep levels steady.

Ulcers: The banana is used as the dietary food against intestinal disorders because of its soft texture and smoothness. It is the only raw fruit that can be eaten without distress in over-chronicler cases. It also neutralizes over-acidity and reduces irritation by coating the lining of the stomach.

Seasonal Affective Disorder (SAD): Bananas can help SAD sufferers because they contain the natural mood Enhancer tryptophan.

Smoking &Tobacco Use: Bananas can also help people trying to give up smoking. The B6, B12 they contain, as well as the potassium and magnesium found in them, help the body recover from the effects of nicotine withdrawal.

Stress: Potassium is a vital mineral, which helps normalize the heartbeat, sends oxygen to the brain and regulates your body's water balance. When we are stressed, our metabolic rate rises, thereby reducing our potassium levels. These can be rebalanced with the help of a high-potassium banana snack.

Strokes: According to research in The New England Journal of Medicine, eating bananas as part of a regular diet can cut the risk of death by strokes by as much as 40%!

Warts: Those keen on natural alternatives swear that if you want to kill off a wart, take a piece of banana skin and place it on the wart, with the yellow side out. Carefully hold the skin in place with a plaster or surgical tape!

Eat near ripe Banana with skin spotted all over.

Beets:

Eat it raw or enjoy as a juice or cook it.

* Protects you from Heart disease
* Protects you from Colon Cancer
* Carrot and Beet juice is a recipe for good health
* Useful in fighting anemia

* Good source of potassium, calcium and vitamin B complex
* Excellent for keeping blood vessels in sound condition
* Drink beet, carrot and Celery juice to beat Arthritis
* Helps weight loss
* Controls blood pressure
* Fights Cancer
* Strengthens bones
Note: People suffering from kidney or gallbladder issues may avoid beets.

Beans:

Beans provide a fantastic option to meat, since they are a great source of protein with least fat. Single serving of dried beans provides 17 grams of protein with only .75 grams of body fat. Actually, the American Cancer Society suggested within their 1996 nutritional recommendations that People in America should "choose beans instead of meat."

Apart from being a great resource of protein, beans really have scrumptious supply of fiber, B vitamins, iron, folate, potassium, magnesium, and several nutrients, and really should be eaten regularly to gain optimal health and wellness. It's suggested that one ought to eat four, ½ cup portions of beans each week.

Beans really are a superb heart healthy food choice. Eating beans frequently is connected with reducing cholesterol levels. Beans, as with other plant-derived protein sources, don't contain any saturated fats, and so are also cholesterol free. Thus, you should limit your saturated fats intake like meat and consume more beans along with other plant protein sources for meat in your regular diet, and you will be on the right path to lowering your levels of cholesterol and enhancing your state of health.

Scientific studies have proven that folate plays a vital role in decreasing the Homocysteine levels. Homocysteine is a compound that could damage the inner walls of our blood vessels if it builds up in your body. Folate reduces this harmful effect by overcoming the Homocysteine molecules. Data reveal that between 20 to 40 % of coronary heart patients have elevated amounts of Homocysteine.

Beans also deliver a potent amount of potassium, calcium, and magnesium. This mixture of electrolytes is connected with reduced chance of cardiovascular disease and hypertension.

It is the plentiful quantity of soluble fiber in beans that appears to help control blood sugar. For those who have blood insulin resistance, hypoglycemia], or diabetes, adding beans to your regular diet can be quite useful to managing your blood sugar. The soluble fiber in beans supplies a slow burning and long lasting supply of energy, composed of complex carbohydrates and proteins for you to make use of.

As these macronutrients take some time for you to utilize, bloodstream sugar levels remain stable. When bloodstream sugar is stable the body does not have to release just as much blood insulin to manage the glucose within the bloodstream. This really is crucial for diabetics, because they, especially, have to control their bloodstream glucose and blood insulin levels to be able to maintain their own health.

As earlier noted, beans really are a wealthy source of fiber. Fiber adds a lot of bulk to meals without adding lots of calories. The reason being fiber is easily digested by our digestive systems. The other advantage is the fact that meals incorporating beans are bulky in character making you feel full without adding calories.

Scientific research indicates that beans might help to prevent certain kinds of cancer, including:

* Pancreatic cancer
* Colon cancer
* Cancer of the Breast
* Cancer of the Prostate

Beans contain both lignins and phytates, which contribute towards the cancer fighting effects of this nutritionally packed super food. Phytoestrogens (that are lignins) are estrogen-like compounds which have been associated with a decrease in the chance of developing cancer of the breast. In addition phytates are compounds which have been proven to lessen the chance of certain kinds of intestinal cancer.

Try eating all kinds of beans, and different bean colors mean that different polyphenols are present. These nutrients have antioxidant qualities and help combat toxins.

Broccoli:

In 1992 an investigator at Johns Hopkins University released his research reports about a compound contained in broccoli that doesn't only prevent the development of abnormal tumors by sixty percent inside the examined group, it further reduced the tumors that did develop by seventy five percent. Broccoli is becoming one of the better-selling vegetables within the United States. In addition you'll find only 25 calories in one cup of broccoli.

Indeed, broccoli which is cruciferous is one of the best food inside our dietary toolbox against cancer. That one factor alone will elevate it to the status as Super food. In addition, broccoli also improves the defense system, cuts down on the incidence of cataracts, supports cardiovascular health, evolves bones, and fights birth defects.

Broccoli is one of the most nutrient-dense foods known at this time around. In ten most frequent vegetables eaten in the U.S. broccoli can be an apparent champion if this involves total polyphenol content. It has more polyphenols than other popular options. Only beets and red onions have over abundance of polyphenols per serving.

The development of cancer in your body is a progressive illness that begins at the cell level and typically only ten to 20 years later is recognized as cancer. While research continues to find techniques for preventing this deadly disease -next to coronary disease the top killer of Americans, most scientists have begun to feel that cancer could be easily prevented than cured.

Weight loss program is the finest tool everybody has at hands to guard ourselves from developing cancer. Everyone knows the typical Western diet plays a substantial role in the development of cancer as we understand that no less than thirty percent of cancers are believed to be caused by our diet habits.

Popular studies point to the role that broccoli plays with other cruciferous vegetables in cancer prevention. One ten-year study, launched with the Harvard School of Public Health, of 47,909 males showed an inverse relationship between the consumption of cruciferous vegetables and the development of bladder cancer. Broccoli and cabbage appeared to provide the best protection. Numerous studies have confirmed this. As way back as 1982, the country's Research Council on Diet, and Cancer learned that "there is sufficient epidemiological evidence to indicate that use of cruciferous vegetables is vital to reduction in cancer."

One study shows that eating about two portions every day of leafy eco-friendly vegetables may result in a fifty percent reduction in the risk for many types of cancer. While all crucifers seem to operate in getting rid of cancer, cabbage, broccoli, and also the Brussels sprouts seem to be the very best. Just half a cupful of broccoli every day will safeguard you from numerous cancers, particularly cancer of the lung, stomach, colon, and rectum. No surprise broccoli is the #1 on the National Cancer Institute's report on super foods. Indeed, eating broccoli or its relatives is similar to acquiring an all-natural dose of chemoprevention.

The key components in broccoli are the phytochemicals, indoles, and the Sulforaphane. These are remarkably potent compounds that fight cancer on numerous levels and raise the enzyme levels that really help get rid of cancer causing carcinogens, and kill abnormal cells. It can help the body limit oxidation-the process that initiates many chronic ailments-at the cell level. Indoles attempt to combat cancer through their effect on excess estrogen. They block excess estrogen receptors in breast cancer cells, controlling the introduction of excess estrogen-sensitive cancer of the breast. The key indole in broccoli-indole-3-carbinol, or I3C-is particularly effective as breast cancer prevention agent.

Researchers estimate that broccoli sprouts provide several times more effective power compare to mature broccoli to counteract cancer causing chemicals in our body. A sprinkling of broccoli sprouts on your salad or perhaps in your sandwich is capable of delivering greater benefit than a couple of broccoli spears. Good news particularly for children-who will not eat broccoli. Check out http://www.broccosprouts.com to understand more about this miracle super food.

This super food is not only a best safeguard against cancer; it has many other good benefits, too.

Broccoli family of veggies (crucifers) is wealthy in folate, and vitamin B, essential and healthy for expecting moms. Some birth defects for instance Spina Bifida are actually connected with folate deficiency. A cup of raw broccoli, chopped in small pieces, provides greater than 50 mg of folate. Folate can also be active in aiding to eliminate Homocysteine within the bloodstream. It is important to avoid elevated levels of Homocysteine as these are associated with heart disease. In addition Folate aids in cancer prevention. Surprisingly, deficiency related to Folic acid is very common and frequent in many parts of the world.

Everybody knows cataracts are very common as we grow old. Broccoli may help here too! Broccoli has ample phytochemical carotenoid anti-oxidants like zeaxanthin and lutein. Both are beneficial to inside of the eye, the retina and the lens. Some studies show that eating broccoli at least 2 times per week reduces the possibility of getting cataracts by 23% , in comparison to people who consumed broccoli only once per month or less. Further any effect to our vision from exposure to ultra violet rays is minimized due to these phytochemicals in broccoli.

These cruciferous vegetables like broccoli are rich in calcium and beneficial to our bones. Raw broccoli has 41 mg of calcium and 79 mg of ascorbic acid (vitamin c), which inspires the calcium absorption. Dairy products on the other hand, normally promoted as source of calcium do not have vitamin c (ascorbic acid) and have more fat and calories compared to 25 calories / cup of chopped broccoli. Also it provides vitamin k supplement, that's essential for blood clotting and in addition, it supplements our bone health.

So in nutshell broccoli provides us the flavonoids and carotenoids, with ascorbic acid, folate, and potassium that really help prevent coronary diseases. Furthermore, it offers plenty of fiber, vitamin B6, and Vitamin E which improves our cardiovascular health. Broccoli along with eco-friendly green spinach, is filled with coenzyme (CoQ10), which is a great fat-soluble antioxidant.

For those who inherit a powerful dislike for the taste of cruciferous vegetables, which could be a bit bitter, may add Sea Salt to improve the taste, or try it as stir-fried with soy sauce or add these veggies to your baked dishes.

Chapter 3- Cinnamon

Cinnamon is really more valuable than a scrumptious accessory for food. Among the earliest spices or herbs known and used in traditional medicinal practices, cinnamon is presently being analyzed for its advantageous effects on a number of health conditions. Indeed, recent findings show particularly its benefits for those who have type II diabetes. That alone has elevated it towards the status of the Super Food (Spice).

Probably the most exciting discovery concerning cinnamon is its impact on bloodstream blood sugar levels and also on triglycerides and levels of cholesterol, all of which may benefit people struggling with type II diabetes. In a single study of 60 patients with type II diabetes, it has been discovered that just consuming half a tea spoon of cinnamon daily for 40 days , fasting serum blood sugar levels were decreased by 18 to 29 percent, triglycerides by 23 to 30 %, low-density lipoproteins (LDL) by 7 to 27 percent, and total cholesterol by 12 to 26 %. Wow, that is nothing to ignore!

It's particularly interesting to note that the benefits of this cinnamon dosage results were effective even up to 20 days after the participants stopped taking it after the 40 day test period.

This indicates that you simply need not eat cinnamon every single day to savor its benefits. The cinnamon by its blood insulin-improving qualities isn't the only spice to exhibit a positive impact on bloodstream blood sugar levels. Cloves, bay leaves, and turmeric also show advantageous effects.

Cinnamon is also known as an antibacterial agent. The fundamental oils in cinnamon can stop the development of bacteria in addition to fungi, such as the common yeast Candida. In a single interesting study, a couple of drops of Cinnamon Oil when mixed with 3 oz. of carrot broth, restricted the growth of bacteria up to 60 days. By comparison, bacteria prospered within the broth without any cinnamon oil. Cinnamon has additionally been proven to work in eliminating the E. coli bacteria.

A current fascinating study discovered that just smelling cinnamon elevated the subjects' cognitive ability and really performed like a type of "brain boost." Future testing will disclose whether this quality of cinnamon could be utilized to avoid cognitive decline or enhance cognitive performance.

Chapter 4- Dark Chocolate

Ever heard the saying "you can have the cake and eat it too!" That is true for chocolate dark or no dark. However it can add calories, if you indulge too much into it as chocolate is 30% fat and 61% carbs. Any way, if you are seeking health benefit then dark is better. It has Polyphenols with antioxidant properties. The research has shown that dark chocolate, because of these properties improves blood flow and helps lower your blood pressure and is heart healthy.

Additional research conducted by Dr. Norman Hollenberg at Harvard Medical School proved that those subjects who drank cocoa with higher amount of flavonol experienced higher amount of nitric oxide activity compared to subjects who drank cocoa with low amounts of flavonol. The higher nitric oxide activity increased relaxation of blood vessels and blood circulation and helped preventing high blood pressure. He also found subjects with high flavonol cocoa had increased blood flow to the brain. Interestingly these polyphenols also inhibit clotting of the blood.

So we have a product which is high in calories due to cocoa butter consisting of oleic acid which is mono unsaturated fat, good fat and stearic acid which is a saturated fat however does not increase blood cholesterol.

As a matter of fact studies have shown that dark chocolate has positive effect on improving HDL the good cholesterol. No wonder it qualifies as Super Food.

Chapter 5- Eggs

I remember days when there was a big scare about eating eggs. There was connection established between eggs and increase in cholesterol levels. We were advised to throw away the yellow part just cook the whites.

I believe nature produces things with proper balance if we consume in moderation. Yellow and white portion in the egg when cooked together and consumed in moderation does not affect cholesterol levels as per new research. The yellow egg yolk contains an essential nutrient called choline, so do not discard the yolk.

As a matter of fact one can consume eggs (one or two) few times a week with great benefit providing great source of protein, vitamins and essential amino acid called Leucine which helps burn fat in your body.

How to Shop For Eggs, In This Ever Increasing Marketing Hype World

In my grocery store they carry Large Eggs AA, small eggs A, Brown Organic eggs, Cage Free Eggs from chickens not kept in cages and are free to roam about and so on.

Each variety is priced different, organic being most expensive.

If you are health minded person and are organic food lover and buy mostly organic food then stay with the organic variety or similar product.

Here are the qualifications for organic eggs. The USDA organic standards are the strictest food production standards in the world. Certified organic farms are required to follow the strict production rules of the USDA's National Organic Standards as per this site www.ams.usda.gov/nop and are regularly inspected by an independent third party for compliance.

Organic hens are allowed access to the outdoors, and never kept in confinement cages, providing many benefits such as better quality of life for the animal, superior animal health, and greater nutritive value in food derived from the animal.

These hens are fed only certified organic feed, grown on land not treated with synthetic fertilizers or pesticides for a minimum of three years.

Organic animals must not be genetically modified and cannot be fed food from genetically modified sources.

In comparison to above Regular eggs are from chickens kept in the crowded cages. They are kept under lights day and night to increase egg production. Beaks and sometimes claws removed. Antibiotics and/or hormones are pumped into the chickens. If you want to be an Egg expert check out this site.

http://www.incredibleegg.org/egg-facts/eggcyclopedia/g/grading

Chapter 6- Flaxseed

Flaxseed is one of the best source of omega-3 fatty acids which are heart healthy. In addition these are a great source of lignins which help protect against breast cancer. Flaxseeds are also rich in fiber, magnesium, potassium, iron and protein. Flaxseed can be purchased as a ready to use flaxseed meal. It should be kept refrigerated once open to keep oils safe to use without going rancid. Of course, you can buy seeds and just grind a small portion just for immediate use in a mini blender like Magic Bullet.

How to Use:

Simply sprinkle 2 table spoons over your oatmeal, cereal, or yogurt. You can add to muffin mix, pancake mix or your bread mix if you bake your own. Just a small quantity, 1 to 2 Tablespoons, consumption per day will give you daily requirements of linoleic acid as omega-3 fatty acid. Flaxseed is also available as Flaxseed oil. Make sure you buy the organic cold pressed variety. Store it in refrigerator.

The late famous doctor Johanna Budwig created a special recipe to defeat cancer using a mixture of flaxseed oil and low fat cottage cheese. This is one of the best recipe even to prevent cancer.

Here is the actual information from their site:

To make the Budwig Muesli, blend 2 Tablespoons of flaxseed oil with 4 Table spoons low-fat Cottage Cheese with a hand-held immersion electric blender for up to a minute. If the mixture is too thick and/or the oil does not disappear you may need to add 2 or 3 Tablespoons of milk. Do not add water or juices when blending flaxseed with cottage cheese. The mixture should be like rich whipped cream with no separated oil. Remember you must mix ONLY the flaxseed and cottage cheese and nothing else at first. Always use organic food products when possible. Next mix in by hand 1 teaspoon of honey.

For variety you may add other ingredients such as sugar free apple sauce, cinnamon, vanilla, lemon juice, chopped almonds, hazelnuts, walnuts, cashews, pine kernels, rosehip-marrow. For people who find the Budwig Muesli hard to take these added foods will make the mixture more palatable. Some of our patients have even added a pinch of Celtic sea salt and others put in a pinch of cayenne pepper for a change.

Note: I have very slightly modified the above procedure to make it easy. Take this sometime in the morning every day or any other time that works for you.

You will be surprised to start seeing results in 4-6 weeks. Do not discontinue. Also since this is a food it should not interfere with your medication but if you are not sure please consult your doctor.

For additional research click on http://www.budwigcenter.com/anti-cancer-diet.php

Caution: Above information is not meant to replace the attention or advice of physicians or other health care professionals.

Chapter 7- Garlic

The famous Garlic with rich sulfur compounds, comes from Onion family. It has been in use from ancient times and its use is often easily detected by its typical pungent flavor around kitchens and restaurants.

Though originated in Asia, it is widely used around the European nations and Africa as well.

It is commonly available as a bulb consisting of individual cloves.

The beneficial sulfur compound allicin is not present in fresh garlic. However when a clove of garlic is either crushed, chewed or cut, this sulfur compound is instantly formed giving it that famous odor and it is also responsible for its medicinal values.

Here are some claims worth making a note about.

Garlic is claimed to help reduce High Blood Pressure

It is also good for treating high Cholesterol

It is said to help regulate blood sugar

It is frequently used to combat cold and cough. Sip on to a hot cup of tea with few garlic cloves, cut into pieces in it.

It has anti-fungal and antiseptic properties as well.

Throughout the ages garlic has been effective for heart health, arthritis, and to avoid cataracts of the eye.

Recent findings are encouraging about garlic to fight cancer, and as anti-inflammatory and antiviral agent.

Apart from Allicin, garlic has potassium, zinc, polyphenols, vitamin B6, phosphorus and vitamin C, selenium which fights heart disease and protects against cancer, and manganese.

No wonder garlic is a real Super Food.

Regular use of garlic, even eating just couple of cloves a day can lower your bad cholesterol, LDL by 10% within a short period of time while improving your good cholesterol HDL and reducing your triglycerides.

In addition one would lower the blood pressure or keep it under control. Further research shows, regular use of garlic decreases the risk for colorectal cancer and prostate cancer.

Garlic also has antibacterial properties and is effective against antibiotic resistant strains such as ciprofloxacin and staphylococci.

Personal note: If you have a tooth ache, chew on a garlic clove. Its antibiotic properties will give you relief until your dentist can see you.

It is interesting to note that some people believe that hanging a bulb of garlic outside the house or place of business wards off evil spirit. It must be that pungent smell! Just kidding.

Looking for Garlic recipes? Check out this site: http://www.garlicrecipes.org

Chapter 8- Honey

Very few people may know the full value of honey. Honey is the only food on the planet that will not spoil or rot. It will do what some call turning to sugar. In reality honey is always honey. However, when left in a cool dark place for a long time it will do what I rather call "crystallizing". When this happens I loosen the lid, boil some water, and sit the honey container in the hot water, turn off the heat and let it liquefy. It is then as good as it ever was. Never boil honey or put it in a microwave. To do so will kill the enzymes in the honey.

Honey contains 180 plus known substances and has antioxidant properties. It is widely used since old times for

* For Respiratory diseases
* Skin diseases
* Urinary diseases
* Eczema and psoriasis
* Dandruff
* Gastrointestinal diseases
* Helps maintain blood sugar levels

* Improves antioxidant capacity of the body
* Honey has ability to inhibit growth of bacteria, fungi and viruses.

Honey also contains salicylic acid, minerals, alpha-tocopherol, and oligosaccharides. Oligosaccharides increase the number of "good" bacteria in the colon, reduce levels of toxic metabolites in the intestine, help prevent constipation, and help lower cholesterol and blood pressure.

The phenolic content of the honey depends on the pollen used by the bees. The color of the honey is a good way to determine its health benefits. Darker the color better the value. For example Illinois buckwheat honey, the darkest honey, has twenty times more antioxidants than California sage honey which is the lightest in color.

There are more than 300 varieties of honey available in North America. Some of the popular ones are Clover, buckwheat, and orange blossom. Just remember dark honeys are more robust.

Caution: It is not advisable to give honey to children younger than 1 year old. Honey may contain clostridium botulinum spores which may cause botulism in infants.

Honey has excellent wound healing properties including first degree burns. The wounds dressed with honey seem to heal quicker due to anti-bacterial properties.

The use of honey increases good bacteria in the colon, improving digestion and help avoid constipation.

Chapter 9- Oats, Onions and Oranges

Oats:

If you are looking for high fiber and protein food, oats fit the bill. However recent research into oat, oat bran or even oat flour has revealed additional excellent information about this super food. It is rich in phytonutrients, lignins and Vitamin E. Low in calories and rich in zinc, copper, and thiamine. A good source of potassium and magnesium and pantothenic acid. The best news is product like oatmeal is served in almost all restaurants serving breakfast. It is very affordable and popular cholesterol, reducer. It is the soluble fiber called beta glucan in oats that is very beneficial. Just a bowl of oatmeal a day keeps your heart healthy! The fiber also helps keep the colon free of toxins including avoiding colon cancer due to special ingredient in oats called Ferulic acid which is a potent antioxidant.

Note: Add ground Flaxseed (Flaxseed meal) and Wheat germ to your bowl of oatmeal at breakfast to stay healthy. Basically a high fiber diet is very helpful in keeping heart healthy, maintain blood pressure and keep colon healthy.

Onions:

This super food is used almost in every food preparation there is out there. It is packed with sulfur containing compounds and flavonoids such as quercetin that imparts yellow/brown color to its skin.

It is part of the garlic family. Like garlic you have to slice or cut an onion to get benefit from its sulfur compound like thiopropanal sulfoxide which is very healthy. But darn it, it does make me cry!

I did find if you cut onion in large pieces and soak in water for few minutes and then chop in small pieces you do not cry! Always let chopped onions sit for ten minutes before cooking to develop its aroma and beneficial effects. Like Garlic, Onions are helpful in reducing high cholesterol and high blood pressure. Onions are also great in reducing risk of colon cancer and evidence out there shows onions may help lower the cancer of esophagus, lung and stomach. When shopping for a good health promoting onion, look for Shallots onions and Western Yellow Onions.

Oranges:

Everyone knows oranges are a great source of Vitamin C. OJ short for orange Juice is popular beverage at breakfast table. Research shows oranges and other citrus fruits are beneficial for heart health and even to prevent cancer, diabetes and more.

Oranges and other citrus fruits are rich in flavonoids and the fruit as whole including skin and pulp is healthier compared to juice. The oranges have hesperidin flavonoids which are antioxidants and have antimutagenic properties which prevent cells from developing cancer and in addition it improves the effect of vitamin c. In addition these flavonoids have ability to reduce possibility of heart attack and stroke. Like apple, orange a day keeps the doctor away!

Then another great source for fiber with richest source of pectin, oranges contribute to heart health lowering cholesterol and controlling blood sugar. Citrus fruits like oranges have been credited with low incidences of cancer as well. Eat the orange as whole and juice the fruit with skin. The peel has this very healthy oil known as Limonene which can slow down tumor growth. All citrus fruits including oranges, mandarins, and lemons contain this limonene in their peel and has ability to help our enzymes stop cancer before it stops.

Tip: Freeze the whole fruit (orange, lemon, etc.). Then once frozen, thaw it for a while, and then cut the whole fruit in small pieces and blend it and eat the pulp and all. You can also use citrus peels in cooking, if you like. However Vitamin C probably will be lost in cooking.

We can write a whole book on Vitamin C, but since we are talking about citrus fruits, we know we have a great source of this vitamin in these fruits. The vitamin C supplements do not provide as much benefit as the whole fruit since the fruits have in addition polyphenols that have the power to protect us against strokes. A recent study for men shows, drinking one glass of OJ daily may reduce the risk of stroke by 25%.

We are so lucky this super food is available in abundance and is very affordable as well. Please take advantage of it.

Chapter 10- Quinoa

Quinoa has become a popular grain among health conscious population. It is gluten free and is 36% soluble fiber and 64% in-soluble fiber and is easy to digest. It is rich in lysine (essential amino acid), unlike wheat and rice, and supplies calcium, magnesium, phosphorus and iron. It has high protein up to 18%, and is a good source of dietary fiber. It has a nice nutty taste when cooked and there are excellent recipes available on the web. Here is a quick link to quinoa corp. website for many valuable recipes and tips.

http://www.quinoa.net/181.html   Here is their basic Quinoa recipe.

The Basic Quinoa Recipe

This light and wholesome grain may be prepared quickly and easily with this basic method. Place Two cups of water plus one cup of quinoa in a 1.5 quart saucepan and bring to a boil. Reduce to a simmer, cover and cook until all the water is absorbed, about 15 minutes. You will know that the quinoa is done when all the grains have turned from white to transparent, and the spiral-like germ has separated. Makes 3 cups.

To prepare in a **rice cooker**, simply treat quinoa like rice. Add two parts water to one part quinoa, stir, and cover. Unlike rice you can stir quinoa a few times while cooking to prevent burning in the bottom of the pan and when the cooker shuts off, the quinoa is done.

Chapter 11- Red Wine

Since early history as far as back as 5000 B.C. red wine has been found beneficial to our health. Now the media has caught up and wine industry has taken a lead in promoting health benefits of red wine.

Here are some well-known facts.

Resveratrol a compound found in red wine has shown results to increase life span and protect against Alzheimer's disease.

Red wine improves digestion, promoting the growth of beneficial bacteria.

Researchers in Spain have found that a glass of red wine per day reduces the risk of Lung Cancer.

Research also shows that certain red wines like Chianti, Merlot, and cabernet sauvignon contain melatonin. This may help you sleep.

Also being an antioxidant it has anti-aging properties.

Red wine has excellent effects on your heart health because of resveratrol and anti-oxidant properties.

Red wine consumption, 1 glass per day, reduces the risk of prostate cancer.

Same is true for Breast Cancer.

People who drink up to 2 glasses of the red wine are less prone to colds.

Resveratrol seems to lower bad cholesterol, LDL, and has anti-inflammatory properties.

Red wine intake reduces the risk of kidney stone formation.

Red wine has anti-clotting effect on the blood.

Moderate consumption, 250ml, per day seems to help hypertension.

Chapter 12- Spinach

Spinach is one of the powerful leafy green vegetable full of long list of nutrients.

Rich in vitamins, minerals, omega-3 fatty acids, glutathione and alpha linoic acid antioxidants to fight against cancer; Carotenoids lutein/zeaxanthin to prevent macular degeneration keeping our eyes healthy. Also rich in chlorophyll, vitamin k and coenzyme Q10 and more keeping our heart healthy.

Spinach is also rich in folate which helps our heart stay healthy reducing dangerous levels of homocysteine to ward off stroke and heart disease.

In addition the spinach is a good source of potassium and magnesium which help in lowering blood pressure.

Spinach can be used in salads or could be lightly cooked in olive oil and seasoned to taste.

Spinach and its twin Kelp go well together and are easily available and very affordable.

Here are some spinach recipes for you.

http://allrecipes.com/recipes/soups-stews-and-chili/soup/vegetable-soups/spinach-soup/

Here is You Tube link for Spinach dip.

http://www.youtube.com/watch?v=YLGfTj5b Nnk

Chapter 13- Tea, Tomatoes and Turkey

Tea is popular in Europe, Asia, Far East, China and India. Its usage is growing in the United States as well. Asian and Chinese restaurants invariably serve hot tea and mostly herbal kind like Green tea.

Common Tea is a black leaf tea available in tea bags (example-Lipton tea bags) that we are so used to dipping in hot water and let it brew until we get the right color. Then adding milk and sugar is optional. Some people prefer a dash of lemon instead and not milk. I am told that adding milk or cream to tea changes its basic chemistry and tea is no longer the tea!

Let us see what Tea has to offer that it is considered to be a Super food before I share with you how to make a perfect cup of tea, the old English way.

1) The phyto chemicals in tea has proven to be very beneficial for our bone health.

Study shows people who have been drinking tea on a regular basis for 10 years or more have stronger bones.

2) Tea also has polyphenols, powerful antioxidants that protect us against damage from free radicals. This improves our chances to ward off cancer and ability to stay young and healthy. In addition tea has immune boosting properties as well.

3) A recent study has shown that people who drank 2 to 3 cups of black tea a day were 70% less prone to heart attacks. Keep your arteries clean and lower your cholesterol by drinking 4-6 cups of tea a day.

4) Did you know Tea has less caffeine than coffee! Almost 3 times less. Just 40 mg per serving (8 oz. cup) compared to 130 mg in 8 oz. of coffee. So next time you are at Starbuck switch to Tea. That extra caffeine can put a dent in your digestive system.

5) The fluoride and tannins in Tea help your teeth and gums stay healthy. Just avoid sugar in tea that does damage to your teeth and gums.

Drinking black tea may be with few drops of lemon juice is a good alternative.

6) Contrary to popular belief, tea could also be hydrating your body, provided you do not consume 5 or more cups of tea at one time. Then the caffeine overload might kick in and cause diuretic effect.

7) Tea could be zero calorie drink if you do not add milk and sweeteners. So if you are watching weight drink black tea with lemon. You can add Green Tea to your diet which has excellent ability to increase your metabolism and help you towards your weight loss goal.

Green tea also contains EGCG an antioxidant which appears to be lot more powerful than many antioxidant vitamins. Black tea has EGCG but is mostly lost in manufacturing process involving fermentation. Hence Green tea is touted for weight loss.

Here is a recipe from Royal Society of Chemistry for perfect cup of Tea.

There seems to be an interesting argument about the right temp. So to speak for tea before you drink it and when to add milk to it. Experts feel adding milk in the cup and then pouring hot water over it and then brewing tea bag adds to the taste.

Read on--

Ingredients: Loose leaf Assam tea (any good brand would work), soft water, fresh chilled milk, white sugar.

Implements: Kettle, ceramic teapot, large ceramic mug, fine mesh tea strainer, tea spoon, microwave oven.

Method: Draw fresh soft water and place in the kettle and boil. While waiting for the water to boil place the ceramic tea pot containing a quarter of a cup of water in a microwave oven on full power for one minute.

Place one rounded teaspoon of tea leaves per cup into this ceramic pot.

Take the pot to the kettle as it is boiling, pour on to the leaves and stir.

Leave to brew for three minutes.

Now the ideal receptacle is a ceramic mug.

Pour milk into the cup first followed by the tea, aiming to achieve a color that is rich and attractive.

Add sugar to taste.

Drink at 60-65C, to avoid vulgar slurping which results from trying to drink tea at too high a temperature.

To gain optimum ambience for enjoyment of tea aim to achieve a seated drinking position in a favored home spot where quietness and calm will elevate the moment.

Tomatoes:

The tomatoes have most powerful antioxidant called lycopene. It is responsible for the color of tomatoes as well. Lycopene has shown positive results against cancer in many studies. It helps protect against skin cancer. Tomatoes also contain high fiber and are a good source of beta-carotene. Harvard medical research study by Dr. Giovannucci in 1995 found that 48000 men surveyed who ate ten or more servings of tomatoes per week had reduced their risk for prostate cancer by 35%. All tomatoes products, sauce and paste are more effective than raw tomatoes. Hence processed tomatoes and cooked tomatoes have lot more lycopene than raw tomatoes.

Evidence shows tomatoes are also effective against breast cancer, bladder and lung cancers. The antioxidant properties of tomatoes are also beneficial for heart health. The men who had lower lycopene levels were more prone to heart attacks according to research conducted by German scientists. The European research established the same results that lycopene was most protective against heart attacks.

Tomatoes are also good source of potassium, niacin, Vitamin B6 and folate. Potassium is effective for maintaining blood pressure, niacin controls elevated blood cholesterol. B6 and folate reduces levels of homocysteine in turn reducing risk of heart disease.

Turkey:

Turkey is not just for Thanksgiving! It is available year round. It very lean protein rich in niacin, vitamin B6 and B12. Thus helpful in keeping your heart healthy and lowering your risk for cancer. It is low in fat and is very affordable. Turkey is high in protein, essential for growth and repair as part of a varied and balanced diet and healthy lifestyle. Nearly all protein found in turkey meat can therefore be used to maintain the function and health of our body cells. Cooked turkey contains 34g of protein per 100g, which is nearly 3/4 of an adult's recommended daily allowance. Turkey offers as much protein as roast beef but without as many calories or grams of saturated fat. There are ton of recipes on turkey on the web. Pick the ones you like. I simply love roast turkey sandwich on rye bread with potato salad and deli pickle.

Chapter 14- Walnuts, Water, Wild Salmon and Wheat

I am a bit nuts about nuts. Granted, nuts do have calories but the benefits of eating handful of nuts like walnuts everyday has proven to cut your chances of getting heart attacks by at least 15%. In addition to reducing your risk for diabetes and cancer Walnuts are rich in omega-3 fatty acids known as alpha linoleic acid, plant sterols that help reduce cholesterol levels, Walnuts also are a good source of fiber and protein in addition to magnesium helping maintain insulin and glucose levels. The copper, folate and vitamin E which has gamma Tocopherol providing anti-inflammatory properties. Vitamin E is also proven, by a study conducted by American Medical Association, to help lower risk of Alzheimer's disease. Walnuts are also rich in essential amino acid called Arginine, which improves the blood flow by making the blood vessels smooth and flexible, thus helping reduce the blood pressure. Adding to the long list are Flavonoids, Resveratrol, for healthy cholesterol and polyphenols like Ellagic Acid for prevention of Cancer.

An interesting old wife's tale, somewhere years ago I read, said that the looking at the shape of some nuts you could tell its benefits: Walnuts look like a brain hence good for memory, Alzheimer's and so on. Almonds are shaped like eyes and are good for your eyes. Cashews look like our kidneys- you get the idea. In any case nuts of all kinds are good for your health.

Here are some recipes from the web. You might like it.

http://www.walnuts.org/walnuts/index.cfm/recipes/

http://homecooking.about.com/od/appetizerrecipes/r/blapp85.htm

If you would like to pursue further information about Walnuts and get to know its benefits and get a bit technical, check this link: http://www.whfoods.com/genpage.php?tname=foodspice&dbid=99#healthbenefits

No wonder Walnuts make the grade to be super food.

Water:

Our body is almost 70% water. Our Tissues and organs are mainly made up of water.

Our muscles are 75% water. Brain is 90% water. Bone is 22% water. Blood is more than 80% water. The functions of water in human body are vital. The water transports nutrients and oxygen into cells

* Moisturizes the air in lungs
* Helps with metabolism
* Protects our vital organ
* Helps our organs to absorb nutrients better
* Regulates body temperature
* Detoxifies
* Protects and moisturizes our joints
* Helps your skin look healthy and younger
* Improves your productivity as brain is 90% water
* Improves digestion and good for relief from constipation
* Reduces the chance of bladder and colon cancer
* Less chances of getting kidney stones

* Great for healthy heart and lung functions

Dehydration causes -Dry Skin, Fatigue, and Hunger, headaches, dark urine and you feel thirsty.

Drink 6-8 glasses of water a day to avoid dehydration.

Drinking water almost costs nothing and is available everywhere. Keeping your body hydrated helps your system perform well at cellular level and further can help you achieve your weight loss goals as well.

Dehydration slows your metabolism and that in turn makes your body store fat. Simply drinking adequate quantity of water every day helps you achieve optimum metabolism.

Drink slowly or simply sip your water. An old saying has some value. Eat your water and drink your food.

Basically drink or sip as if you are eating. When you eat your food eat slowly and chew slowly until the food feels like liquid or watery and then drink it.

Fruits rich in water like water melon and fruit juices also count towards hydrating your body. Coconut water for example is great for hydrating your body and is rich in beneficial electrolytes as well.

Wild Salmon:

As we all know fish has been promoted heavily as healthy food providing us with good fat so to speak known as polyunsaturated fats. I bet you, fish oil and capsules are heavily promoted and are widely used by many people and more so with the older men and women. The fish provides us with both valuable Omega -3 and Omega-6 poly unsaturated fats that are proven to keep our heart healthy and reduce our chances of cancer!

All Salmon varieties are not created equal. When shopping for it or ordering at a seafood restaurant ask for Wild Salmon. There are 2 varieties basically, Farm raised and Wild.

The farm raised salmon is raised in small crowded ponds near the ocean where they are subject infections.

To avoid diseases these crowded fishes are treated with strong antibiotics which in turn show up in the fish meat when we cook.

Instead of eating natural food source while swimming freely in the wild ocean, these farm raised variety is fed dry fish food which is often laced with cancer causing agents or other unhealthy curing agents. Then to add to our insult this variety is fed with artificial pigment to give fish the natural looking pink color that the wild salmon gets naturally feeding in the wild. That should be illegal.

Hence the farm raised variety has much less omega-3 fatty acids and more of omega-6 which we do not need as much, as we get enough of it.

The wild salmon is the richest source of omega-3 fatty acids. Preparing fish at home is one of the easiest dish. Just buy fresh wild salmon, marinate it for half an hour and put it on the grill. It cooks fast and cook it medium and enjoy with side of greens. Avoid breaded and deep fried recipes.

It is important to note that most of our foods like corn, sunflower and cottonseed oils are rich in omega-6 fats, hence most of us get enough of omega-6. However for best health we need a good balance between omega-6 and omega-3. Recommended ratios are within 4:1. In reality we get lot more of omega-6 compared to omega-3.

To correct this imbalance and to benefit most from these two healthy fats to stay in correct ratios we need to increase our intake of omega-3. That is where wild salmon comes to our rescue. Consuming wild salmon four or more times per week would help and is recommended.

Many other benefits from eating fish are getting DHA acid that is vital for our eyes and for avoiding macular degeneration. Salmon also provides you protein.

It is also interesting to note that our brain is 60% fat. These omega-3 fatty acids help regulate brain's activity including mood changes, memory and our nervous system.

If wild fresh Salmon is hard to get where you are look for other cold water fish, like sardines and trout or opt for canned Alaskan Salmon. Always watch for mercury content in the canned fish and sodium.

Here are some varieties of wild Salmon you may come across.

Sockeye salmon: Rich, moist, and firm, Sockeye salmon flesh enjoys a reputation as the reddest of the wild pacific salmon species. Its robust and rich comes from its high oil content which makes it ideal for canning and hot and cold smoking. Second to king salmon (Alaska) in Omega-3 fatty acids, Sockeye is an excellent heart-healthy food.

Coho Salmon: Favored among smokers for their reddish-orange color and high oil content, Coho salmon have a taste somewhere between Chinook and Atlantic salmon. Its heart healthy Omega-3 oil content color ranks third behind Chinook and Sockeyes.

Fresh Atlantic salmon: Red to pinkish meat, Atlantic salmon is moist and oily. The taste is delicate and is excellent source of Omega-3 fatty acids, which have been proven to be great for the heart. The fish is also favored by many smokers for the quality of product it allows.

Copper River Salmon: The **Copper River** or **Ahtna River** is a 300-mile (480 km) river in south-central Alaska in the United States. It drains a large region of the Wrangell Mountains and Chugach Mountains into the Gulf of Alaska. It is known for its extensive delta ecosystem, as well as for its prolific runs of wild salmon, which are among the most highly prized stocks in the world. It is the tenth largest river in the United States, as ranked by average discharge volume at its mouth.

Because the Copper River salmon's journey is so long, these fish must store extra fat and oils in order to survive the long trip. This high fat and oil content is why Copper River salmon are recognized as some of the world's best eating salmon.

Here are some recipes for preparing wild Salmon dishes at home.

http://www.recipesearchup.com/recipesdownload/index.php?promo=wild%20salmon

Wheat:

Does not matter what country you visit you will find wheat products in use as a staple food. The inner part of wheat kernel before any processing is done , known as wheat germ is loaded with protein, fiber, folate, vitamin E, thiamine, vitamin B6, magnesium and selenium, iron and zinc. In addition wheat germ is great source of omega-3 fatty acids.

You can simply sprinkle wheat germ on cold or hot cereal or mix it in a blender with your favorite smoothies. Mix it with pancake mix and muffin mix and so on. Just 2 tablespoons of this product per day will give you 4 grams of protein and 2 grams of fiber. **It is effective in reducing cholesterol.**

Wheat products like wheat bread does have carbohydrates. However you have to look at the whole package. Wheat has that outer rich layer called the bran full of nutrients and fiber, then the middle part contains protein and carbohydrates with vitamin B, and the wheat germ the inner layer full of vitamin B-6, vitamin E and several nutrients mentioned earlier here.

All these components as a whole have life enhancing health benefits.

When whole grains are refined into white flour the nutrients like bran and wheat germ are destroyed leaving behind protein and carbohydrates. When buying bread or wheat products avoid the ones made from refined wheat or grains. Products made from whole grains have much better health benefits and it is proven that it further reduces the risk of Cancer as well.

Grains and Cardiovascular Diseases: Whole grains are also heart healthy. A nine year study conducted involving more than 34000 postmenopausal women showed that the mortality rate dropped up to 19 percent among women who ate whole grains every day.

Grains and Strokes: A similar study among the group that never smoked and consumed 2-3 servings of whole grain everyday showed 50% reduction in the risk of strokes and 30% lower risk for heart disease.

The whole grains are a natural source of vitamin E and are effective in reducing the risk of stroke.

Grains and Hypertension: Whole grains play a very important part in the diet to stop hypertension. Please refer to http://www.nhlbi.nih.gov/health/public/heart/hbp/dash

It is the fiber in the whole grain that helps blood pressure especially the diastolic reading, lower or bottom number of the two BP readings.

Whole grains contain folate helping lower homocysteine levels which is a risk factor for stroke and cardiovascular diseases.

Individual Concerns: Allergic Reactions to Wheat

Please review this website which is a not for profit organization. It has some very valuable data on whole wheat and towards the end it discusses wheat allergies.

http://www.whfoods.com/genpage.php?pfriend
ly=1&tname=foodspice&dbid=66#healthbenefi
ts

Looking for world of recipes? Check this site:

http://www.whfoods.com/recipestoc.php

Chapter 15- Yogurt

Yogurt was discovered as a result of neglect. Upon finding that goat's milk left in a clay pot in the sun had turned into a strange semi-solid, imagine the courage it took for a person ten thousand years ago to taste it.

It is very interesting to note that any diet or weight loss plan these days talks about cleansing the system. Then they talk about digestive system and probiotics. Probiotic means' for life" basically good for healthy life style.

One of the best source of probiotics is Yogurt especially low fat or no fat variety as long as it has active live strain of healthy bacteria. When shopping for yogurt look for these "live and active" cultures on the label. In addition look for calcium and vitamin D. Look for brand "Fage" which is a "strained" Greek yogurt. Thick and creamy.

This is an age old remedy. I personally know in our family we always prepared homemade yogurt from a sample culture from yogurt made on previous day. Simply mix the culture in low fat milk and then bring it to boil. Then let it cool and ferment overnight. Store inside a covered container or simply inside a microwave oven over night. Make sure Microwave is off and stays off. In the morning milk should turn into thick yogurt. Then you can move it to refrigerator for later servings.

You can also buy from your grocery stores ready to eat yogurt with live strains of healthy bacteria. Avoid flavored varieties due to added sugar. Just plain yogurt would do. Do check the label for live and active cultures.

Yogurt Is Super Food Because It Has

More protein than milk. Almost 9 grams of protein per 6 oz. serving. It is rich in calcium helping bone-mineral density. A single cup of yogurt has 400 mg of calcium and only 100 calories. Great super food to eat to prevent osteoporosis. Do take vitamin D in addition to help absorb calcium. Some of the yogurts in the market do include additional vitamin D.

Yogurt is rich in potassium and in combination with calcium helps maintain healthy blood pressure. Harvard school of public health conducted a study of 5000 university graduates and found that 50% reduction in risk of developing high blood pressure for those who eat 2-3 servings of low fat dairy (milk) per day. They believe yogurt will have same effect

The beneficial bacteria in yogurt fights Diarrhea. Many antibiotics when taken affect digestive system in a negative way and often causing Diarrhea. Yogurt if taken regularly will help offset the effects of antibiotics. In any case if you are taking antibiotics and experience Diarrhea, increase your intake of yogurt.

Unfortunately your doctor prescribing these antibiotics do not even recommend benefits of yogurt. Most of them routinely advise us to avoid dairy products!

Research has shown recently that yogurt even helps reduce cholesterol and improves our immune system and can be helpful in eliminating ulcer and gastric cancer.

Probiotics in Yogurt help in relieving symptoms of IBS. In addition helping inflammatory Bowel Disease.

The probiotics in yogurt also help maintain healthy skin and nasal passages and help keep healthy digestive track.

There is strong evidence that probiotics in yogurt help as cancer fighting agent particularly so for colon and breast cancer by reducing inflammation and stopping the growth of cancer causing micro flora in the intestine.

Yogurt has ability to stimulate our immune system. Research has proved that yogurt can effectively reduce the common pathogenic bacterium-Staphylococcus aureus thus improving the immune system.

Yogurt seems to help women prone to yeast infections which is common in women who are diabetics. The active culture in yogurt helps reduce the vaginal pH and bring to normal, 4.0 to 4.5.

Try eating yogurt as a snack between meals and avoid hunger attacks. It makes you feel full.

So you have it! Yogurt with all these health benefits works synergistically and promotes our health in so many ways. No wonder it is a super food since ancient times.

Yogurt making tips: Here is good link to start.

http://articles.chicagotribune.com/2012-03-28/features/sc-food-0323-prep-yogurt-20120328_1_yogurt-bacteria-lactic-acid

Chapter 16- Conclusion

Visit My Other Kindle Publications

1) "Herbs and Spices for Health and Healing"

http://tinyurl.com/kq74nlf

2) Pain Treatment with Magnets: Read Actual Case Histories. [Kindle Edition]

http://tinyurl.com/n4ak2mj

3) E D T A -This Four Letter Word May Save Your Life [Kindle Edition]

http://tinyurl.com/n7r7ge6

Thanks.

Prem